AUTISM
AND THE STRESS EFFECT

of related interest

Supernourishment for Children with Autism Spectrum Disorder
A Practical Nutritional Approach to Optimizing Diet for Whole Brain and Body Health
Angelette Müller
ISBN 978 1 84905 383 9
eISBN 978 0 857007 46 9

Reframe Your Thinking Around Autism
How the Polyvagal Theory and Brain Plasticity Help Us Make Sense of Autism
Holly Bridges
Foreword by Stephen W. Porges
ISBN 978 1 84905 672 4
eISBN 978 1 78450 177 8

Autism Movement Therapy (R) Method
Waking up the Brain!
Joanne Lara with Keri Bowers
Foreword by Stephen M. Shore
ISBN 978 1 84905 728 8
eISBN 978 1 78450 173 0

AUTISM AND THE STRESS EFFECT

A 4-STEP LIFESTYLE APPROACH TO TRANSFORM YOUR CHILD'S HEALTH, HAPPINESS, AND VITALITY

THERESA HAMLIN

FOREWORD BY DR. TEMPLE GRANDIN
AND DR. JOHN RATEY

Jessica Kingsley *Publishers*
London and Philadelphia

Bristol Stool Chart on p.226 is reproduced with kind permission
from Dr KW Heaton, formerly Reader in Medicine at the University
of Bristol. © 2000 produced by Norgine group of companies.

First published in 2016
by Jessica Kingsley Publishers
73 Collier Street
London N1 9BE, UK
and
400 Market Street, Suite 400
Philadelphia, PA 19106, USA

www.jkp.com

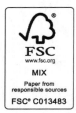
FSC
www.fsc.org
MIX
Paper from
responsible sources
FSC® C013483

Library of Congress Cataloging in Publication Data
Hamlin, Theresa.
Autism and the stress effect : a 4-step lifestyle approach
to transform your child's health, happiness
and vitality / Theresa Hamlin ; foreword by Temple Grandin and John Ratey.
pages cm
Includes bibliographical references and index.
ISBN 978-1-84905-748-6 (alk. paper)
1. Autism--Psychological aspects. 2. Stress
(Psychology) 3. Diet. 4. Exercise. I. Title.
RC553.A88H3518 2015
616.85'8820651--dc23
2015018549

British Library Cataloguing in Publication Data
A CIP catalogue record for this book is available from the British Library

ISBN 978 1 84905 748 6
eISBN 978 1 78450 178 5

Printed and bound in the United States

This book is dedicated to the staff at The Center for Discovery who give of themselves tirelessly to support and enhance the lives of our children and their families.

CONTENTS

FOREWORD

Dr. Temple Grandin & Dr. John Ratey

Autism is a broad spectrum and there is a huge shortage of information to help individuals with the most severe complex forms of autism. Many of these individuals remain nonverbal, lack basic daily living skills and may have destructive behavior. Many behavior problems are caused by being in a constant state of stress due to the "noise" of sensory over sensitivity.

This insightful book describes a multi-pronged approach of correcting health problems that contribute to disruptive behavior, lots of exercise, and behavioral methods. Careful use of medication is also part of the program.

Parents and teachers who work with older children and adults with severe autism, who are either nonverbal or only partially verbal, should read this book.

Dr. Temple Grandin, Author
The Autistic Brain
Thinking in Pictures

Stress can be harmful for all of us, but especially for those with other underlying problems like autism spectrum disorder (ASD). Stress becomes particularly toxic when it doesn't end; this creates an inner world of what I call "noise." In this state, the best of us cannot pick out the relevant data from the background, and are often in a non-stop panic state that is a booming, buzzing confusion. From my perspective as a psychiatrist, it is one of the most important concepts to understand and navigate in the treatment of autism.

It was at the start of my career, almost 35 years ago, that I had my first exposure to patients with ASD and their reaction to stress. They were severe, adult cases, exhibiting aggression and self-abusive behavior. Patients were often heavily drugged, misdiagnosed as having everything from schizophrenia to manic depression, and housed in chronic mental hospitals. Witnessing and breaking down the destructive behaviors exhibited in such an un-healing environment led me to writing a paper called "The Concept of Noise." It recognized that aggression and self-abusive behavior in the autistic brain is frequently a nonverbal expression of internal stress. The paper not only theorized a new way of looking at ASD behaviors, it also led to my lifelong relationship with Temple Grandin. Temple is famous for giving voice and articulating what it's like to be inside the mind of someone with ASD. While attending one of her lectures in Boston, Temple quoted the "Concept of Noise" paper, confirming a "noisy brain" is a good description for the autistic brain, especially under any kind of stress. Temple has been instrumental in my continual learning and understanding of what might be going on in the brain and feeling state of autistic individuals, with stress leading to more confusion, more uncertainty, and more noise.

We now know if the noisy state is unrelenting, for a number of reasons, it is difficult, if not impossible, for change, healing, and progress. From a biological perspective, when toxic stress is reduced, there is an increase in the brain's neuroplasticity, the necessary tool to learn and retain new information and behaviors. If we don't take the important steps of reducing the high stress levels most ASD people find themselves experiencing, learning compensatory and situationally appropriate behaviors and strategies becomes overwhelming, with frustrations erupting in meltdowns and what we used to call "catastrophic reactions." This increase in internal disorientation not only generates aggressive, self-abusive, self-stimulatory behaviors, but also flight or internal withdrawal. These uncontrollable behaviors are both heartbreaking and frustrating for families, caregivers, and those living with autism, no matter where they may be on the spectrum.

If there is anywhere in the world examining and employing best practices for reducing internal stressors and noise, it is The Center for Discovery (TCFD) in upstate New York. Headed by Patrick Dollard, an internationally recognized thought leader in the field, TCFD cares for hundreds of developmentally disabled students, including 250 individuals living on the extreme end of the autism spectrum. Many of them are nonverbal or struggle to communicate as well as having difficulty with self-care. For over 30 years, Dr. Terry Hamlin has taken the leading role in overseeing the groundbreaking programs, research and therapeutic tactics employed by TCFD. While treatment norms for ASD in the past have usually consisted of the basics of medication and behavioral therapy, TCFD has developed a revolutionary, all encompassing holistic approach geared specifically to the ASD individual. With her experienced and caring staff, Dr. Hamlin has been at the forefront of finding the best ways to lower negative stressors, while at the same time, building on coping mechanisms, introducing new, healthier behaviors, and employing methods to make it all stick. Impressive results have been achieved by going beyond the pharmaceutical and behavioral fixes, incorporating and recognizing concepts often overlooked or under-utilized in the treatment of ASD; the importance of proper diet, the contribution of adequate sleep, the benefits of exercise and movement, the positive results of being in nature, all while aiding those with ASD in improving their interaction and connection

The important work coming out of TCFD is being initiated, researched, and backed by some of the world's foremost authorities in these specific areas. While attending my first meeting on campus, I looked at the conference table of experts gathered by Dr. Hamlin, and recognized it as something akin to an autistic NASA project. Brain scientists specializing in sleep, diet, nature, movement and exercise, and more, travel on a regular basis from Harvard, MIT, Northeastern, Columbia and Georgia Tech, to the grounds of TCFD, seeking out solutions to tackle the major challenges associated with autism. The work continues, but there is already so much we know. With her rich experience, practical knowhow, and commitment to educating others, Dr. Hamlin is the perfect messenger to open the door to the newest and most effective treatments. Her book serves as an important and practical guide for families, caregivers, and those living with Autism.

While Dr. Hamlin and The Center for Discovery handle only the most difficult cases, the revolutionary treatment methods researched, individualized, and employed by Dr. Hamlin should be followed by everyone anywhere on the spectrum, leading to a more connected, self-regulating, fulfilling life.

By reading these pages, things can only get better.

Dr. John J. Ratey MD
Associate Clinical Professor
of Psychiatry at Harvard
Medical School

ACKNOWLEDGEMENTS

This book is the product of years of experience and teamwork with professionals, parents, the Board of Directors, and staff at The Center for Discovery, New York. Under the dynamic and passionate leadership for the past three and half decades of Patrick H. Dollard, CEO and President, friend and colleague, The Center for Discovery has become recognized for the highest quality of care and treatment for those with complex disabilities. The staff continually challenge themselves to discover new solutions to some of life's most challenging problems. They are selflessly dedicated and motivated to help others.

I would like to recognize Glenn, Evelyn, Terri, Susan, Trina, and Amy who not only encouraged my writing of this manuscript, but also provided critical expertise and commentary from their experiences as parents of children with autism.

I would also like to acknowledge expert Chef Cesare Casella for his fierce dedication to quality food for all of our guests who live at The Center. He has masterfully brought the farm to the table with his team of da Vinci Chefs.

And lastly, I thank my husband, Kelly, who has gone to sleep many a night to the sound of my typing. Without his support, I would not have completed much of what I have set out to do in my life for helping children.

INTRODUCTION

This book is revolutionary and timely in its message as it transforms a highly complex condition and distills it into an understandable 4-step approach toward transforming your child's health and vitality. The four steps include understanding and learning to regulate the child's environment, eating and nutrition, emotional self, and energy expenditure. It offers a hopeful and positive lifestyle approach that can help the whole child and the whole family. By whole child I mean not only from an educational perspective, but from the medical and psychological perspectives as well—body and brain.

The purpose of this book is to teach parents and those who support children who have autism how to increase health and vitality by decreasing stress on the body and brain so that the children can heal, learn, and advance to their greatest potential.

After many years of educating, treating, and supporting children with autism and working with their families, I am compelled to share what my colleagues and I have learned. It is my hope that this book will restore common sense to a world that is wrought with fear, anger, confusion, and sadness as parents struggle to find the right supports and treatments for their children. It's no longer acceptable for professionals to treat only the observable core symptoms of autism. One must look below the surface, into the child's biology, to find solutions to what may be one of life's most devastating conditions currently affecting our children. The implications of not finding new solutions are beyond comprehensible. As the numbers of children diagnosed with autism continue to rise every minute of every day, autism now affects 1:68 in the United States, which is at least 1 percent of the world population. This rate is growing annually by 10–17 percent, reflecting the beginnings of a worldwide epidemic.

This easy-to-read book proposes a new framework for intervention that is based in science, practical, understandable, and free to parents. It is our hope to create a better future for children and families affected by autism. It offers an empowering lifestyle approach and a way of thinking about autism that doesn't currently exist in the mainstream. Part 1 gives us insights into the problems seen in children who have autism, where stress was highlighted as a major problem affecting all areas of functioning. Part 2 is devoted to understanding the key components of life that can cause or calm a stress response in the child and how you can regulate or adjust those components to minimize, avoid, or eliminate the stress response. That's what this book is about— learning to actively and consciously regulate our experiences and affect change. The last two chapters (Part 3) are about how parents and those supporting children with autism can collect valuable information, and how they can use that information to regulate and guide their decisions and inform others.

This approach works, as evidenced by the hundreds of children and families already helped through this framework. It's a success story that must be shared—parents should not have to live feeling isolated, shedding tears that come from an unfathomable world where hope dwindles as time passes. It's time to rewrite the story for children with autism and their families, and that's exactly what *Autism and the Stress Effect* does.

PART 1

Chapter 1

A NEW WAY FORWARD

This chapter will share struggles of parents as they try to help their children who have complex forms of autism, along with successes from parents who have discovered new ways to help their children. The evolution of autism that led to modern day treatments will be explored and the chapter will end with a proposed new way forward for families and children and those supporting children with complex forms of autism. By complex forms of autism, I mean those children who struggle with communication or may even lack the ability to talk; those who have limited self-help skills and may need assistance to even get dressed in the morning; those who often have no real friendships; and those who may exhibit maladaptive behaviors. Although this book is written for parents and professionals supporting these children, there is a wealth of information that is just good common sense for all of us living on this planet especially if we find ourselves living with a lot of stress. I urge you to take from this book what you think will help you, your child and your family the most.

SHARON

While on my way home from a meeting with a group of parents who were worried about their children's transition to adult life, my cell phone rang. I picked up the phone not recognizing the number. "Hello." There was a pause, and then I heard her voice.

"This is Sharon," she said. I knew immediately who it was. "You probably don't remember me, but we met at a wedding about 10 years ago. I was there with my husband and son, Anthony."

"Of course I remember," I said. What I didn't say was that I had a hunch she would call someday.

"Oh, good," she said. "Do you have a minute? I have a question." I pulled over, and began to listen to her story.

Anthony had a severe form of autism, which was evident when I first saw him playing under the table at the wedding where we met. He wasn't able to communicate or socialize at all. At that time Sharon, like most parents of very young children with autism, was committed to keeping Anthony in her local school. She was volunteering in Anthony's classroom to make sure he was getting the right services. After school, she arranged for a small army of people to help continue his education well into the evening hours. On weekends, she managed to get volunteer college students to help carry out his program. Sharon was committed to curing Anthony's autism.

I could hear a level of desperation in Sharon's voice. "I didn't want to call you, but I wasn't sure who else to call. I've exhausted all my resources, and I just don't know what to do next." Sharon shared with me a few months later that calling me meant defeat to her, admitting that despite all her efforts, her son wasn't getting better. These are moments that are most humbling to me. Parents should not have to get to a point of feeling defeated.

"Tell me what you need," I said. This wasn't the first call like this that I had received, as a matter a fact, there have been many calls like this one over the years from parents who had tried every treatment imaginable, and just didn't know what to do next for their children. Initially, the best response is to just allow parents to talk, and that's exactly what I did.

Sharon told me that she had lost her job and was on the verge of losing her husband. As she described, Anthony was out of control and was becoming very aggressive toward her and his little sister. He was a big boy at 13 years of age and very strong. The school he was in couldn't handle him, and were encouraging her to find another. She really needed advice from someone who had experience with children with more complex forms of autism. Sharon remembered our conversation at the wedding, and knew that I worked in a place that focused on children with severe autism. She talked for over an hour. She cried, and said that she hadn't slept in years. It was apparent that she found some relief in speaking to me as she knew I would understand and I was connected to other parents who had experienced similar situations. She needed confirmation that she wasn't as alone as she felt.

Having a child with a more complex form of autism, one that significantly interferes with communication, socialization, and daily routine functioning, is really challenging. There are fewer resources available, less information about these children, and the demands on families are relentless. After listening to Sharon, I was able to make several calls to find supports in her area that could help. Anthony really needed a comprehensive psychiatric and medical workup by doctors who understood the complications associated with autism, followed by a development of new program interventions, and intense training for those supporting him in how to help.

At The Center for Discovery we evaluate hundreds of children like Anthony, providing assessment, interventions, training, and education for children, families, and professionals. It's a comprehensive integrated approach, and one that is highly successful for most children and their families.

BILLY

In December 2013, a newspaper article appeared in the *New York Daily News* about a boy who had apparently been saved from a life of isolation and perhaps worse as reported by his father.

We first met 16-year-old Billy in his home. He was diagnosed with severe autism. Along with his diagnosis, Billy was obese at 280 lbs, and he demonstrated severe aggressive and harmful behaviors that terrorized his family. Billy ate mostly pizza and cheese and had irregular bowel patterns. He didn't attend school because of problems in the school environment. Thus he stayed at home refusing to leave the safety of his bedroom. His sleep and daily rhythms were totally erratic.

According to his father, on some days, Billy would suddenly go berserk and destroy the whole house. The police would have to come to restrain him. Billy's father and his mother would clean up the mess and weep. "We would weep, not for ourselves. For him. For Billy. We didn't know how to help him," said Billy's dad to a news reporter. Billy had a complex form of autism that significantly affected his ability to interact with others and interact in his environment. Eating, getting ready for school, participating in class, and making friends were all severely challenging for Billy and his family.

Unfortunately, many parts of Billy's and Anthony's stories are similar to what many parents experience when they have a child with a more complex form of autism. We often hear from parents that their child with autism is not sleeping or they have aggressive behaviors, their diet is highly limited to processed foods, and they may have gastrointestinal or other immune problems. Each situation is unique, but they all share many of these common problems.

After six months of attending the program at The Center for Discovery (The Center), Billy's father stated that his son Billy had been saved. He told a reporter for the New York Daily News who was following Billy's story that the professionals at The Center had transformed his overweight, unhappy, violence-prone son into a trim, joyful and productive young man. "On Thanksgiving, we took Billy to my cousin's house and he ate with perfect table manners, using a knife and fork," his father stated. "Billy ate responsibly, and when he was done, he asked to be excused" (*New York Daily News* 2013).

A year and a half later, Billy is happy and thriving with friends. He is taking control of his life and holds a job that has meaning to him and to his coworkers who depend on him. He still requires ongoing organizational support, but there is collective knowledge now about what helps him to be calm, healthy, productive, and happy. Most importantly, he is loved and he is lovable. He has friends and those who want to be his friend; he is moving forward on his journey toward achieving his greatest potential.

The rethinking of Billy's treatment for his autism began with speaking to his parents and the people supporting him. There was much dialogue around what was causing his unhappiness and violent behaviors. The team began to understand that these problems were not fixed—they were being influenced by key factors occurring in the environment and by Billy's poor health. Strategies were then implemented to help him regulate the enormous amount of stress he was experiencing on a daily basis. Slowly but surely, he began to feel better and his behaviors began to decrease—he was happier and more content and willing to interact. The intervention, as explained in this book, is a lifestyle, one day at a time approach that makes a remarkable difference. It requires new thinking and new ideas.

The condition of autism exists at increasingly higher rates with very few treatments to alleviate all of its difficulties despite the billions of dollars spent and the countless hours given for behavioral treatments. Billy is just one of hundreds of children transformed by an approach that seeks to understand all the problems that are entangled in the complexity of autism. Billy was "saved" according to his family because his family and those supporting him learned to regulate the essential components in his life. Now Billy is on a journey toward regulating his own life.

This book is a new way forward, where my colleagues and I will share knowledge, insights and methods used to transform the Billys in the world of autism. Take a moment to imagine as a parent of a child who has autism being with people in a place that focuses on knowing more about the root causes of the problems detected in children with complex autism: a place where top scientists, researchers, physicians, educators and clinicians all come together to better understand how to support children with autism and their families; where health is studied in relation to behavior; where food is considered an important component of health; and where sleep, exercise, and daily rhythms are seen as primary to learning, functioning, health, and vitality—a place that observes, lives, works, and plays with the children day in and day out, and never rests. Such a place exists at The Center for Discovery and it is located in New York State on 1500 acres of farm landscape in the foothills of the Catskill Mountains.

Fortunately, as the science around autism has progressed and more information and knowledge has been accumulated, there are a growing number of likeminded people in the field with more places being developed with similar philosophies.

The Center has been caring for and supporting families and children with complex needs for more than six decades. We have developed a comprehensive system of care that is unique and thoughtful, and informed by science and research. The program was born out of a world where children were failing in typical public school and community settings and parents needed alternatives. The Center staff knew that if they were to help these children and their families, they needed to find new ways of thinking and helping—new models of care and intervention. Failure was not an option—the system needed to change. This book will reveal what has been learned—the foundational principles developed to begin supporting children with complex forms of autism.

If you are a parent, grandparent, educator, clinician, or physician of a child with autism, then this book is for you. It brings together new understanding from practitioners who are studying human health with the experts in autism, who understand how chronic disease and biological problems are affecting those with autism.

Before exploring a new way forward, in this chapter I will explain why there is a need for that new way, beginning with the current state of autism, followed by a historical review of how we developed the current framing of autism, and then ending with a new way of thinking about autism that has led to new interventions.

Chapters 4 through 7 will provide a view into the world of children with complex manifestations of autism. A clear vision will be shared of how to begin to help these children regulate their environments and experiences so that they can be successful, feel better, and ultimately reach their greatest possible potential. It is not a panacea or a one-size-fits-all method. This method recommends a lifestyle approach where each child is recognized as an individual living in a unique and dynamic environment. The four essential components, which include environment, eating and nutrition, emotional self-regulation, and energy regulation, are meant to be flexible and responsive to each child and family. The chapters contain suggestions and strategies to implement these components at home, in school, and in community environments.

This first chapter will begin by introducing the facts about autism—what we know today including current statistics about the unexplained increase in the number children diagnosed. Rooted in the observations of those who first discovered and put a name to this condition, Chapter 1 will reframe how to think about autism.

THE DIAGNOSIS OF AUTISM

The population of children affected with Autism Spectrum Disorders (ASD) is seemingly growing at a very fast pace. The current prevalence in the US is 1:68 children, and 1:42 boys (CDC 2014). Studies in Asia, Europe, and North America suggest autism affects 1 percent of the world population, and that number is increasing. A study in South Korea reported prevalence of 2.6 percent (Kim *et al.* 2011).

The US IDEA Data Accountability Center Report identified 401,416 children aged 6–20 with more complex forms of autism who were receiving services in schools. According to the report, there are probably many younger children not yet counted who will eventually be added to this number (Dufault *et al.* 2012). Dufault noted a 91 percent increase in the number of children with ASD receiving special education services in the US between 2005 and 2010. It would appear from these statistics that autism is the fastest growing disability ever experienced in world history.

Highly controversial, however, is whether there actually is an epidemic of autism or whether the rise in numbers of those diagnosed is simply an artifact of better identification. Gernsbacher, Dawson and Goldsmith (2005) made the case in the article, "Three reasons not to believe in an autism epidemic," that a broadened diagnostic criteria coupled with greater public awareness accounted for most of the assumed increase. However, for those of us trying to help parents and schools support these children, the argument is moot. What we know is that there are thousands upon thousands of children and families worldwide who need help. For those of us who are trying to help, the only thing that matters is that we offer the right support that they need now.

According to the Centers for Disease Control (CDC), autism is a lifelong neurodevelopmental disability. If you are a parent or someone working in the field, it should come as no surprise that there is a huge range of uniqueness among children with autism including differences in onset and nature of the condition as well as severity of the symptoms. It's been said by many in the field that if you've seen one child with autism, then you've seen one child with autism, which illustrates the diversity in the symptoms. That being said, I would like to suggest that if you were to examine the medical profiles of all children with autism, you would begin to see patterns of symptoms that are similar, regardless of the severity. The medical symptoms are revealing, as you will see in the next set of chapters, and should be guiding many of our treatments.

The profound rise in the number of children identified, along with the complexity of symptoms, has unfortunately left the public education systems and the medical community seriously under-prepared and under-trained in diagnosis, assessment, and treatment of these children who have a broad array of challenging conditions. Unfortunately, there is no medical test at present to diagnose autism; rather, a diagnosis is made through observation of the child and an interview process with the parent or support personnel by a skilled clinician. This process is not an exact science as it relies on human judgment. Autism occurs in all racial, ethnic, and socioeconomic groups, and is five times more likely to occur in boys. I have traveled the globe and the problems are the same—children and families are struggling and desperate for answers. The professional community is underprepared, but almost every professional I meet is highly motivated to know more in order to better help children and their families.

The new DSM 5 criteria for diagnosing autism

The Diagnostic Statistical Manual (DSM) 5, the most current manual (American Psychiatric Association 2013), is used to diagnose autism spectrum disorders (conditions) and other mental and behavioral disorders. In the past, there was a triad of problems identified and noted separately. DSM IV separated out social and communication deficits into distinct categories. The fifth edition released on May 18, 2013 offered a collapsed definition of autism spectrum disorders/conditions that includes two primary domains: (a) persistent deficits in social communication and social interaction; and (b) restricted and repetitive patterns of behavior. And, of great concern to many individuals who identified themselves as having Asperger's Syndrome, the new DSM 5 eliminated the diagnosis of Asperger's and included it as part of the autism spectrum.

In the new DSM 5, individuals with ASD must demonstrate significant problems in social-emotional reciprocity (the back and forth of social engaging that happens between people), deficits in nonverbal communicative behaviors used for social interaction (facial expressions and body language), and deficits in developing, maintaining, and understanding social relationships. Individuals must also demonstrate at least two types of repetitive patterns of behavior including: stereotyped or repetitive motor movements; insistence on sameness or inflexible adherence to routines; highly restricted, fixated interests; hypo- or hyper-reactivity to sensory input; or unusual interest in sensory aspects of the environment. These problems are judged in terms of their severity by an expertly trained clinician or physician. If the child is determined to meet criteria based on observation and interviews with the parent/support personnel, they are labeled as having autism within a range of severity ranging from one to three.

THE EVOLUTION OF AUTISM

The story of putting a name to autism began in the 1940s when Austrian born psychiatrist Dr. Leo Kanner first began to notice that a small group of his patients were presenting with seemingly similar, yet highly unusual types and patterns of behaviors. These children were unlike any others he had encountered in his practice. He was puzzled by the children's lack of responsiveness to others, especially their parents. He began to intensely study these 11 children, meticulously documenting his observations and finally describing in a seminal paper what he called, "Autistic Disturbances of Affective Contact."

Kanner borrowed the term autism from Eugen Bleuler (1950), a Swiss psychiatrist. Autism means "autos" from the Greek word for self, which has been interpreted to mean "isolated self." Bleuler began using the term autism in 1911 to refer to patients who possessed symptoms of schizophrenia. Kanner, however, was convinced that the behaviors he was observing were not indicative of schizophrenia, but rather a completely separate condition. His work formed the basis of today's study of autism.

In Kanner's (1943) groundbreaking paper, "Autistic Disturbances of Affective Contact," he described 11 patients documenting their uniqueness and their commonalities.

> This is from the start an extreme autistic aloneness that, whenever possible, disregards, ignores, and shuts out anything that comes to the children from the outside. Direct physical contact or such motion or noise as threatens to disrupt the aloneness is either treated as if it weren't there, or if this is no longer sufficient, resented painfully as distressing interference. (p.242)

Kanner used descriptor words such as "autistic aloneness" and presented autism as a problem of the child wanting to be alone and not able to handle the social world: a child who would become stressed and anxious at the "threat of interaction." These descriptors were subtleties, yet commonalities documented throughout his 11 observations. They have been integral to our understanding and treatment of autism, as his paper describes children struggling to function under highly stressful conditions. The result of chronic stress on the brain and body can severely impact health and vitality, and must be attended to and treated effectively.

Kanner continued to further describe the anxious tenseness that he observed in the children, which he felt was a result of the uneasy anticipation because of a possible interference of others. It appeared from Kanner's descriptions that it was the threat of the uncertainty of human interaction that triggered the stress or anxious tenseness in the child.

> Objects that do not change their appearance and position, that retain their sameness and never threaten to interfere with the child's aloneness are readily accepted by the autistic child. He has a good relation to objects; he is interested in them, can play with them happily for hours. (p.246)

> Tricycles, swings, elevators, vacuum cleaners, running water, gas burners, mechanical toys, egg beaters, even the wind could bring about a major panic...Yet, it is not the noise or motion itself that is dreaded. The disturbance comes from the noise or motion that intrudes itself, or threatens to intrude itself, upon the child's aloneness. (p.245)

In this description one can see that it is not objects that are source of the child's stress, but it is intrusion of the object and or the human interaction that results in stress.

Kanner continued, "The dread of change and incompleteness seems to be a major factor in the explanation of the monotonous repetitiousness and the resulting limitation in the variety of spontaneous activity" (p.246). Once again Kanner describes the constant threat or panic that the child experiences with the thought of change. The need for sameness using objects in a repetitive way appeared to be the child's way of trying to maintain a body and mind in homeostasis and a state of calmness—balancing the stress and threat conditions perceived through human interaction, which according to Kanner, were fraught with uncertainty and unpredictability.

Kanner's 1940s lens influenced by the theoretical framework of his time without today's advances in medicine and science, gives us thoughtful insights about the now highly prevalent condition we continue to call autism. His fundamental emphasis on the child's need for sameness and the contentedness the child demonstrated when alone and with objects is not too far from our daily observations of the children we initially meet.

The children who come to us often have been expelled from public school or are on the verge of expulsion; are without friends; have perseverative or idiosyncratic interactions with objects in the environment; and may or may not have language. Some possess basic social interactions and some do not, but all of these children exhibit high levels of tenseness and stress, and all are described as being highly anxious by their parents and support givers.

Kanner astutely noted that there was an "anxious tenseness" when children with autism were in the presence of others. Today we can measure that "anxious tenseness" using technology to measure the child's internal physiological state and cortisol in blood serum to measure the body's reactive state, confirming Kanner's initial observations. Kanner brilliantly illuminated the fundamental problem that is most concerning in many children with autism today: they function under chronic stress conditions.

A word about Asperger's

During the same era as Kanner, Dr. Hans Asperger was discovering another "autistic psychopathy" in children at the University Children's Clinic. The subset of children he identified had normal intellect but expressed extreme difficulty, paired with anxiety in social settings. According to Asperger, their self-absorbing interests and lack of what he described as "empathy," dominated their social interactions. He called the condition "autistic psychopathy" and described it as marked by social isolation. He referred to his patients as "little professors" because they appeared to have knowledge in a variety of specific areas well beyond their age. Based on findings from current research, the children with this form of autism are known to react more strongly to stressful situations than their peers as evidenced by an increased heart rate and abnormal EEG measures. A study conducted by Gaigg and Bowler (2007) demonstrated abnormal fear and anxiety in these children. It should be noted that with the adoption of the new DSM 5, these children who were once labeled as having a separate and distinct condition, Asperger's Syndrome, are now considered part of the autism spectrum.

We now have an understanding of how autism was originally identified and framed. Since that period of time there have been many scientific advances and more research about the effects of autism on a child's biology and ability to interact. The following section will explore some of those advances and set the stage for a fundamental new framing of intervention for those with autism.

AUTISM TODAY

In the paper "The concept of noise," Drs. Ratey and Sands (1986) described children with autism and other mental health conditions as experiencing an internal state of crowding and confusion created by a variety of stimuli, the quantity, intensity, and unpredictability of which make it difficult for the child to tolerate and organize their experiences (p.290). They called this concept, noise. They found that stimulus overloading occurred in the child's brain, particularly when the stimuli were unpredictable or uncontrollable. This type of stimulus was similar to those that could derive from human interaction. These stimuli could produce internal chaos, impulse actions, impaired functioning, and increased physiological stress. Insisting on sameness with an atmosphere of low-level irritation was a way that the child could manage the threat of becoming overwhelmed.

In a study, Temple Grandin, Ph.D. (1984) described that her nervous system was under constant stress, and she was always in a state of hyper-vigilance. She suffered from "nerve attacks" and continuous "stage fright." As she aged her anxiety attacks worsened, destroying her ability to function and causing serious stress-related health problems. Dr. Grandin was a strong supporter of vigorous exercise and other stress-reducing techniques including psychopharmacology to reduce her stress and increase her ability to function during the day. There will be more about her work in later chapters.

Anxiety and continued stress in children with autism may be the most debilitating problem in the diagnosis, and may profoundly change the outcome for the child for better or worse depending on if it is recognized and how it is treated. Unfortunately, stress and anxiety are not included in the criteria for diagnosing children with autism. They may not even be discussed among educational and clinical professionals treating the child as a possible factor in performance; and they are rarely discussed as a critical biological health problem. Most treatments today are focused on increasing socialization, communication, and school behavior. What is often overlooked is the idea that without addressing stress, these goals cannot be actualized. The only way children will thrive is with a program that takes into consideration the full breadth of their problems and provides interventions to address all of them.

Recent research suggests that anxiety-related concerns are among the most common presenting problems for children with autism (White *et al.* 2009). Fear and anxiety appear to occur at higher rates in children with autism than in their typically developing peers (Kim *et al.* 2000; Leyfer *et al.* 2006). In a recent study measuring physiological stress, Corbett and colleagues (2012) found that children with autism showed enhanced and sustained stress in social situations that worsened with age. In a study that looked at physiological and behavioral stress during a routine dental visit, Stein and colleagues (2014) found that the children with autism exhibited far greater distress compared to their peers without autism. The stress resulted in behavior management problems, which often included the use of restraints. Personal narratives from individuals who have autism communicate lives led in constant fear of any triggers that may result in the "fight or flight" response (Grandin 2006; Jolliffe, Lansdown and Robinson 1992; O'Neill 1998; Williams 1996).

With all of these scientific studies and personal accounts demonstrating similar results, what is being done to address the chronic anxiety, stress, and fear in the child diagnosed with autism? How are we educating and supporting parents as they struggle to help their children at home, in the community, and at school? Unfortunately, it appears that much of this research is not reaching the masses of educators and other professionals supporting the child and family.

It has been my experience that parents know very little about the debilitating problems of stress. Even more importantly, they have little knowledge and few resources for how to regulate and control stress exposures for their children. Parents are quite good at expressing the stress they intuitively see and feel in their children, but they are not given strategies and knowledge about why this exists and how to help. It also appears that very few programs and interventions have been designed to specifically address the core problems of stress and anxiety in children with autism. And for certain, there are only a handful of programs that aim to decrease stress as a way to increase health and vitality in children with the goal of increasing functioning and happiness in children with autism.

What parents don't say

Autism is a complex condition. It is expressed differently in every child and in every family. Because of its complexity, you cannot assume you know the child or the family based on the diagnosis. Each child and family is an individual who is shaped and regulated by the environment and their experiences.

"Tell me about your child" are the first words I say when a parent tells me that their child has autism. Upon initial interviews with parents of children with autism, they almost always describe their child as very stressed or anxious, especially when faced with uncertainty or change in their routine. These are the same descriptors that Dr. Kanner used to describe the children he observed. The stress of the child, as described by parents, can affect the entire family, keeping them up night after night feeling exhausted, frustrated, and even hopeless at times.

I find it peculiar that I don't hear the parents say that their greatest challenges are the lack of eye contact, trouble with organizing, or lack of social-communicative behaviors. It's not that the children do not present with these hallmark traits. They do, but these do not seem to be the problems that plague the family the most. It's almost always the stress result that interferes with and disrupts the functioning of the child and the family: stress that can result in severe maladaptive behaviors and significant negatively spiraling health problems.

An example of this issue can be illustrated in the experience of Bonnie, the mother of a teenage boy. Bonnie described an afternoon with her son when he wanted to go to the diner in town, then to the local market, followed by the car wash, and lastly to see the Jack Russell Terriers at a friend's house. But when the plan for the day was not exactly what he wanted, his behaviors escalated and he became aggressive. He started to scratch and tried to pull Bonnie's hair. Just the slightest change in what he expected caused him to become distressed ending with a series of very serious behaviors that interrupted the entire plan for what was to be wonderful day together with the whole family. The stress caused by the unpredictability of these behaviors was what plagued Bonnie and her family the most.

Before autism was prevalent

During the past decade, there have been many inspirational books written about autism that have provided insights into the complexity of this condition. Many of these books have included case-specific treatments where a few children have experienced a total elimination of autism symptoms. Unfortunately many of these treatments do not have the same curative effect when replicated on great numbers of children with the condition. The treatments are typically aimed at just one symptom of what we now understand is a highly complex condition. The symptoms of autism are not only confusing for parents and professionals; they can be very challenging and frustrating to manage.

Long before autism was prevalent, my colleagues and I were pioneers in a world with a poorly understood population of children with complex and multiple disabilities. Our commitment, as we saw it, was not to institutionalize the care and support for these children as had been done in the past, but to seek new knowledge and understanding about the root causes of the problems we were seeing. We wanted to treat the children's problems so that the children would be healthier and more resilient.

This work required careful observation and an integrated approach to medical and clinical diagnostics to unravel the co-occurring conditions and problems seen in the children. Our committed team of highly skilled clinicians worked together for decades to solve these compound problems, and to create methods to help future generations of children with similar diagnoses and conditions. Our successes have been remarkable. These children are now living in good health and spirit well beyond what anyone imagined just a few decades ago, and their families are happy and peaceful unlike the families who came before them.

A NEW WAY OF THINKING

It may take us decades to fully understand or we may never fully understand all the complexity in the diagnosis of autism, which is why understanding how to prevent added stress on the child is fundamental. As with other complex conditions, autism isn't something that the body has—it's something that the body does as a result of its experiences. Subsequently and fortunately for us, that means there is something that we can do to help.

Together with my colleagues, we offer a commonsense approach with strategies for regulating and/or controlling a child's environment, interactions and experiences as a way to reduce autism symptoms, especially the stress and anxiety that the child experiences from their environment and interactions with others. It's about healing the child's brain and body and decreasing the stress-related symptoms of autism.

It is important to be able to regulate certain key factors in a child's world as a way to control the outcome of the stress effect in autism. It's empowering to know that it is possible to effect change by manipulating certain features of the environment during a child's day. It's also important to realize that life is dynamic and things can change subtly or drastically from day to day. What we are looking for are the bigger changes that most often are seen over time—month-to-month and year-to-year.

The central chapters in this book set the stage for understanding the critical elements necessary to make a positive difference.

The main lesson I have learned about children with complex conditions is that you can't just treat what is observable—the obvious core symptoms of autism; you must look below the surface to the root causes of problems, deeper into the biology of the child, to find solutions. Looking deeper, beyond the core symptoms, is the subject of this book. It is a meant to be a primer for parents and program personnel from which they can build to further a child's learning and happiness.

Chapter 2

FROM INTUITION TO CUMULATIVE KNOWLEDGE

What began as intuition from years of practical experience has now been supported by science. This book has been developed with a unique lens from which to view the relationship of health and the problems most commonly cited in autism. I have outlined the essential components of a program: ones that are foundational and critical in helping children with autism regulate their thinking and responses to their environments. These essentials should help to decrease the stress and ultimate wear and tear on the children's bodies and brains. The approach is safe, practical and easily learned with growing evidence and science to support its efficacy—in other words, it works!

In this chapter, I will share stories from past experiences with programs that serve children with autism. These stories will illustrate why we need to rethink some of our common practices in treating children with autism and their families. These stories will frame the stress effect and autism as experienced by children when professionals aren't aware of the underlying problems that affect the children's ability to function.

EXPERIENCE WITH CHILDREN WHO HAVE AUTISM

For many years I have had the privilege of observing, teaching, and treating children with multiple, complex disabilities including children who have autism, not just in the classroom or clinical setting, but also in a progressive, highly regarded continuum of care model which includes a residentially-based program. It's a program intentionally designed to carefully observe, listen, document and attend to a child's every need and problem; a program that has successfully supported and educated thousands of children and families over the years.

Because I have had the advantage of time with many children who have autism—seeing them in hundreds, if not thousands of different situations, with different people at different times of the day, in different environments—it's evident to me these children are quite resilient and capable of getting better. However, they are also very vulnerable, and often misunderstood and misrepresented in literature and in society at large. Unfortunately many educators and professionals are not trained and skilled in looking for medical problems or other co-occurring problems in autism. These educators are struggling to support these children in their classrooms with little help from the scientific community and few strategies that are proven to be successful.

STEVEN'S STORY

For years I have been educating children with complex conditions, but it was when I met Steven and subsequently hundreds more children like Steven that I felt compelled to write this book in the hope of making life better for those who have autism and for those who support them.

A while ago, I was asked to observe a child for possible admission into the program at The Center. I arrived at Steven's private school and was greeted by an enthusiastic social worker who brought me to Steven's classroom. There were eight children with autism in the class, and all had 1:1 aides supporting them. The teacher was working directly with Steven as he was setting and unsetting the empty table for four—a discrete trial lesson.

He appeared to be engaged in his work without noticing me sitting directly in front of him. The other children and staff also continued working without seeming to notice my presence.

Steven was 14 years old, tall for his age and significantly overweight. His teacher wore earplugs while working with him, and there was a packet of Oreo cookies sitting on the table. The cookies were apparently being used to reward Steven every few minutes for not engaging in what was described as being a deafening screeching behavior. Steven's screeching was apparently so disruptive that the previous behavior plan called for the teacher to abruptly squirt Steven in the face with water to get him to stop screeching. Squirting a child in the face with water, referred to as "misting," is no longer acceptable in our State as it is considered aversive. According to Steven's behavior plan, if he was extremely disruptive he was to be brought into a separate padded room for time out until he calmed down. But, in the meantime, he was to be rewarded with Oreos for being quiet.

During my one-hour visit, Steven stayed on task for about 20 minutes and six Oreos given in halves, but after 20 minutes I was privy to why the school could no longer handle Steven. Beginning with a quick, but penetrating scream aimed at the teacher's plugged ear, Steven began to screech. The screeching intensified for about a full minute and finally he reached out and hit the teacher's arm. Two aides immediately responded as though they had been waiting for the incident. Steven was escorted out of the classroom, thereby ending the session, and causing genuine upset in the entire classroom of staff and children.

I interviewed his teacher, who lamented that the Oreos and Diet Coke reward plan was not working. According to the school psychologist who developed the plan with information from his parents and school staff, Oreo cookies were Steven's highly preferred motivator and the only thing likely to keep him under control. The Diet Coke was added because he liked soda, but the teacher was concerned about Steven's weight. Over time his medication, known for the side effect of weight gain, and his reward plan of Oreo cookies were stacking up against him. Steven was in a negative downward health and behavioral spiral. He was on the verge of expulsion or worse, potentially being sent to an inpatient psychiatric center for adults with mental illness.

I share this story because it is a common one for so many children who seek help today. Additionally, it's not only the rigid educational programs that are problematic. Children with autism often have a combination of health issues as well including gastrointestinal problems, compromised immune systems, trouble sleeping, seizures, anxiety disorders, and metabolic disorders. When combined with poor diets and essential vitamin and mineral deficiencies children's health and ability to function are affected. Autism is the least of their complications. The other medical and health problems are often more immediate and urgent concerns. If not treated, these issues will worsen over time. Professionals need to do more than just acknowledge these problems. Interventions should be examined relative to their effects on the child's overall health and well-being.

CHILDREN WITH MORE COMPLEX SYMPTOMS OF AUTISM

In spite of their sometimes challenging behaviors, these children can be socially appropriate with a wonderful and witty sense of humor. They can engage with measured and sustained eye contact. They enjoy having friends, and are capable of learning and progressing when provided with carefully measured supports and experiences. This understanding, however, can be overlooked for children like Steven. They are often thought to be behaviorally disordered children with psychiatric problems, and sometimes considered to be hopeless and harmful by society. Parents will sometimes tell us that medical professionals have told them to place their child in an institution and move on with their life. Much research and education is needed in order to help children with autism and their families; however, because of the highly challenging behaviors often seen in children with more complex forms of autism, these children are frequently excluded from clinical and research settings. There is still very little scientifically documented information about these children who present with more complex symptoms. School personnel and parents of children with autism unfortunately are often struggling without the much needed support and guidance on how to help and intervene.

In my 33-year career, I have listened to hundreds of parents' experiences. Many have shared their daily struggles of trying to help their child find peace and happiness while simultaneously seeking balance in their own lives and the lives of their other children. Raising a child who has autism, especially a child with a more severe form of autism, is extremely difficult and can be lonely and frustrating. Each day can be different and very demanding. The situation for the child and family can actually worsen during the teen years. The system of supports available to parents needs more practitioners who understand the breadth and complexity of the problems of the child and the resulting problems for the family as a whole.

WHY WE NEED TO RETHINK AUTISM

A second article about Billy appeared in the *New York Daily News* in 2014 with renewed hope from Billy's dad. "I want people who have autistic kids to know that there is hope," he said. This was a new thought for Billy's dad, who just a few years back was hopeless. Now he said he knew better—children with severe forms of autism can get better.

"This weekend, I'm going up to visit my son Billy. He graduates high school on June 17th. Like every other regular high school graduate this weekend, he's got a senior prom date." Billy's dad tried to hold back tears of pride according to the reporter.

On Saturday, Jack and his wife, Jane, drove up to The Center. Billy greeted them, saying he'd already enrolled in night classes in English and country music at the local community college. He showed his parents his world where he does important and rewarding work.

That night the family watched Billy—a child who had torn their New York City house asunder—stride with tranquil confidence across the old fashioned barn-dance floor. Dressed in a tuxedo, Billy led a lovely young woman in a beautiful pink prom dress onto the busy dance floor in the season of spring as the program that saved Billy's life blossomed after the long snows of winter.

Then as the Beatles' "Here Comes the Sun" played, Billy led Jody in a dance to life.

"We stood on the sidelines, wiping tears of joy," said Billy's dad. "Our Billy was no longer 'different.' Billy was like every other American high school graduate this month dancing with a date at his senior prom. How do you ever thank the people who gave your kid a life?"

"You dance," said Billy's dad. Every child and every family should be able to dance—to experience success and happiness. This is the reason we need to rethink autism—so every child and their family can experience joy and happiness in their lives.

In order to help children with autism, I suggest beginning to think differently about autism using an approach that helps to regulate core features of living and interacting that are affected by autism. I hope to impress upon you that children with autism have a lot going on internally that's highly affected by what's happening externally.

Autism is a system-wide problem. It is for this reason that it is important to use a holistic approach for treatment, and also likely the reason that we have not yet found one cure. When a child presents with autism, they do not just experience one or two symptoms; rather, they often exhibit multiple problems.

It's well documented, but not well understood, that children with autism suffer from a whole host of chronic problems such as brain and body inflammation, gastrointestinal and metabolic problems, seizures, sleep problems, high levels of chronic stress and anxiety, general dysregulation of the emotional and physiological body systems, and immune and autoimmune problems—just to name the most commonly cited problems.

A large-scale Harvard study was conducted to examine the medical problems occurring in 14,000 individuals with autism (Kohane *et al.* 2012). The authors confirmed that there existed a large number of medical problems that were occurring at the same time that went well beyond those routinely managed by the pediatricians. They concluded that these conditions require broad multidisciplinary management and remediation on many levels to restore the body and brain to a healthy state.

While the Harvard study was being conducted, Schieve and colleagues (Schieve *et al.* 2011), from the National Center on Birth Defects and Developmental Disabilities, conducted a study that included 41,000 children aged 3–17 years, of which 5469 had one of more of five disabilities including autism, intellectual disability, attention deficit hyperactivity disorder, learning disability, or other developmental delay. It was determined that these children had higher than expected rates of all of the medical conditions that were studied including 1.8 times greater incidence of asthma; 1.6 times greater incidence of eczema; 1.8 times of a food allergy; 2.2 times of frequent, severe headaches; 2.1 times more likely to have three or more ear infections; and 3.5 times more frequent diarrhea or colitis. One note of particular interest related to gastrointestinal problems was that children with autism were twice as likely as children with ADHD, learning disability, or other developmental delays to have had frequent diarrhea or colitis, and 7 times more likely to have experienced these gastrointestinal problems than were children without developmental disabilities. Gastrointestinal problems will be discussed later in this book in Chapter 5 on eating and nutrition.

In a third large-scale study by epidemiologist Lisa Croen (2014) of Kaiser Permanente, more than 2.5 million records were examined. The records included 2108 adults with autism who were compared to 21,080 non-autistic adults. The results of the comparison revealed that adults with autism suffered from the following higher rates of medical conditions than peers:

* 24 percent higher gastrointestinal disorders

* 42 percent higher hypertension

* 50 percent higher diabetes

* 69 percent higher obesity

* 90 percent higher sleep disorders.

The adults also had conditions in the area of mental illnesses that were much greater than their peers such as:

* 117 percent higher anxiety

* 123 percent higher depression

* 433 percent higher suicide attempts.

The adults with autism also had higher rates of less common conditions such as eating disorders, injury from falls, vision and hearing impairments, osteoporosis, and chronic heart failure. The only exception was cancer, which appeared equally distributed amongst all patients—autism and non-autism. Notably, this study revealed that the problems seen in children with autism don't go away as the child ages into adulthood, and can actually worsen. These problems must be recognized, diagnosed, and treated early on or children will suffer the consequences. This requires a whole new system of awareness and management. According to Croen, many adults with autism can become socially isolated, which can interfere with good nutrition, diet, and exercise, all of which further negatively affect medical and psychiatric health. Unfortunately, but not surprisingly, there was also an identified lack of preventive care in the adults who were isolated.

IN PURSUIT OF NEW TREATMENTS

My motivation to better understand the problems in autism has been fueled by battling some professionals who think that the child with autism is defined by their observable behaviors—a biter, a flapper, a runner, or a severely aggressive child—as I've heard children being referred to using these descriptors repeatedly over the years. I have heard from education and medical professionals who have given up on their children, causing parents to give up hope. Some parents have even expressed that their children are intolerable, and I have seen an increased number of children who have been placed in lifelong psychiatric centers and in forensic facilities.

In 2008, a prominent practitioner told me that treating autism from an integrated, health prospective was unjustifiable. He argued that the only viable researched treatment for autism was behavior therapy. He said the treating autism from a whole body approach was like treating a cancer patient without using chemotherapy. He strongly supported a very narrowly focused, rigid behavioral approach, which he likened to chemotherapy for autism. The approach was made up of discrete trail training for rote learning of basic concepts that included food rewards for correct responses. Rewards included M&Ms, pretzels, and potato chips. Staff dangled these foods on their belts in clear Tupperware containers meant to entice the child to behave correctly. It was a program where staff members wore long-sleeved shirts, arm guards and spit shields to protect themselves from the children. Clipboards used by staff were filled with volumes of "+" and "–" marks and they followed the child for all waking hours as though the child was oblivious to this intense level of constant scrutiny.

This was a program where staff and children oozed stress and lacked joy as daily crisis loomed heavily in anticipation of a child becoming uncontrollable: a program that permitted and used seclusion and multiple restraints as a matter of course to control behaviors. Staff believed that children with autism lacked theory of mind, understanding, and feeling and could simply be trained to behave using food as treats and punishment.

In my opinion, this myopic approach for treating autism, focused on treating only the obvious, observable behaviors with operant conditioning, which was dismissive of the child's intellect, health, and humanism.

While I find that this is a narrow approach, it is not totally without merit. Programs that offer positive supports, structure, and organization are quite helpful and supportive of the child's need for external regulation to be successful in their lives. I am deeply concerned, however, about programs that are too narrowly focused, ignore health problems, use seclusion and restraints, and dismiss the intellect of the child with autism.

There is reason for all of us supporting children with autism in the school environment to be concerned as the use of seclusion and restraint as a method of treatment for children with autism appears to be commonplace in our schools. According to the United States Senate report from the Health, Education, Labor and Pension Committee (2014), it was well established that the use of seclusion and restraints including chemical, mechanical, and physical restraints was widespread. Reportedly only 19 out of 50 states had laws providing meaningful protections against restraint and seclusion for all children, while 32 had laws for children with disabilities. And even among the small number of states who limit the use of restraints, only 13 limit the use for emergencies such as life-threatening physical harm. Most concerning is that only 18 states require that the school notify the parent about restraints and seclusion if required for their child. One can only imagine how devastating it could be for a nonverbal child to be restrained or secluded by adults in school and then go home to parents who have no idea what happened to them during the day. Restraints and seclusion in my opinion are the last resort to be used when all other interventions, treatment, and strategies fail in a particular incident. They should not be a permanent strategy in a behavioral plan, but should be viewed as an emergency intervention that necessitates the entire team including the parent coming together to reanalyze the child's program.

It was reported that 70 percent of the reported cases of restraint use in the United States were for children who have disabilities including autism. And it was concluded that, "even if the children suffer no physical harm as the result of the use of seclusion and restraints, studies have shown they remain severely traumatized and may even experience post-traumatic stress disorder" (p.9). Even without this report, it should be quite apparent that we need to find a better way to help our children who experience restraints and seclusion. That will only come once we better understand the particular problems each individual child is challenged with.

I am advocating that the thinking about autism be re-examined. The negative behaviors need to be seen as a symptom of something that is not right in the environment or in the child's biology that must be discovered and treated. The behaviors cannot simply be managed using candy or restraints. We need to discover the root cause(s) of the problems and develop strategies to remedy or regulate the problems.

For an example, I saw data on one of the children who we were screening for our program during my visit to the highly restrictive program previously referenced. The child had a high frequency of aggressive behaviors that occurred typically when he hadn't had a bowel movement for many days. The child was obviously severely constipated and most likely his colon was enlarged and overstretched. He couldn't speak, and could only express pain through hitting and biting. The selected treatment for him when he became aggressive was seclusion and physical restraint. Perhaps that could be considered the right treatment if the goal were only to remediate the observable outward aggressive behavior. However, if the child were treated for hypo-motility of the gut and constipation, perhaps the behavior problems would decrease or go away all together. The child would then readily participate in activities because he actually feels better. Children can't begin to learn if their biology has gone awry—if they are sick, in pain, or in a perpetual state of being overwhelmed.

In the case of the child mentioned above, The Center made the determination to admit him into our program. After several months of regulating his experiences such as how to participate with others and regulating the environment by visually organizing and structuring his activities, and with treatment for his biomedical problems, his major behaviors subsided. His diet of healthier foods, communication ability, and daily functioning significantly improved. He made friends and began to thrive, a response which has continued to the present. This book will explain our approach to treatment and what you can do at home to help your child function and feel better.

There is so much more to learn, but one thing I know for sure is that using rigid, narrowly focused models with negative reinforcement, restraint, punishment, and primary food as rewards is not sustainable or acceptable long-term treatment for anyone, let alone for a vulnerable child who is not healthy.

Chapter 3

EXPLORING AUTISM AND STRESS

This chapter will define what is meant by "the stress effect," exploring what can trigger a stress response in the child with autism and what the body does in response to stress. The science of the stress response is presented so that it can be easily understood by parents and other non-medical professionals. The chapter ends with how parents can help themselves and their children to be successful by enlisting the help of others in their lives.

IS AUTISM A FIXED CONDITION?

Is autism a fixed, psychiatric, behaviorally-based condition? Billy's story makes the case that the problems seen in autism can be regulated, influenced, shaped, and ultimately changed for the better. According to Norman Doidge (2007), psychiatrist and author of *The Brain that Changes Itself*, the past presumption about autism was that it was a brain problem. Traditionally professionals separate the brain from the body. Psychiatry and psychology have rightfully played the lead role in designing the treatments for what had been traditionally considered a brain disorder. However, we now have a better and more thorough understanding that autism is much more than a brain problem. The body or biology problems may be far worse in terms of their negative impact on the child than the problems considered brain related as noted in Chapters 4 to 7.

According to Doidge it was the parents of children with autism who were first to begin to describe the physical and medical problems their children were experiencing. Problems included in their list of concerns were gastrointestinal, bowel, and issues with sleep. Doidge noted that it was apparent that children with autism had inflammation throughout their bodies indicative of brain and body problems.

There has been mounting evidence from clinical studies that Doidge's claims are accurate (Courchesne *et al.* 2011; Gupta *et al.* 2014). With this information, there comes the question of what can be done to alleviate some of the medical problems and the associated stress on the body to ward off the negative effects of early chronic disease. Interventions should be developed aimed at reducing these problems and subsequently reducing the stress effect.

How can we help children feel better and function on healthier levels? I propose that we rethink autism as a condition that can be regulated and improved. In this book, I have done just that by conceptualizing a robust, comprehensive, and integrated framework that seeks to alleviate stress and positively support health and learning by regulating the child's external and internal world. Before discussing the program, let's look more closely at what parents and professionals need to understand about many children with autism.

TAKING A CLOSER LOOK AT THE PROBLEM

This section will focus on stress and particularly what is meant by the term chronic stress and the effect of chronic stress on the body and brain.

Chronic stress, as a result of multiple combinations of problems in autism, turns out to be a potential major culprit in the day-to-day functioning of the child and also in long-term health outcomes (Corbett *et al.* 2009; Naviaux *et al.* 2013). For the past several years at The Center, we have been examining the stress response in children and staff in the classroom during the typical school day. In addition to observing, we are also using technology to capture information about the child's experiences through physiological measures and audio/video recording. In combination, these technologies help to measure the stress levels of children with autism who are primarily nonverbal or have limited language capabilities.

The idea of using physiological measures, which has been studied for decades, is now becoming more commonplace with technology that is more readily available. Three popular objectives measures include the galvanic skin response, heart rate, and body temperature. In their study, Kushki *et al.* (2013) used these three measures and discovered that there are critical differences in the stress response between children with and without autism. The most important finding was that children with autism in the study had increased heart rates at baseline during routine tasks; although both groups stress responses increased during a stressful task, it was the children with autism who demonstrated the greatest and most abnormal responses to stress conditions. It was also found that the children with autism who had higher IQs had a more severe and prolonged stress response. This is important because children with autism, whether they have higher IQs or not, may not always be able to express their feelings of stress, and may not even be aware that they are becoming overly stressed. Children with higher IQs are at risk for a more severe response.

Sometimes you hear from parents and teachers that the child seemed to go from zero to 60 in just a matter of a minute. What they are describing is that the child appeared to be perfectly calm and then just seemed to explode. What needs to be understood is that these children really aren't at zero. They are at higher speeds from the beginning even if we aren't able to visually observe this internal state. This happens because the resting heart rate of some children with autism is higher during normal functioning in comparison to children without autism: to get to a stress level that is reactionary is much faster for some children with autism. We have seen children in our program who appear to be sitting calmly while the teacher is presenting a lesson and then all of sudden the child will jump up and start to run. What the teacher cannot see, but what is visible to our research staff, is that the child's stress level is elevated and something seemingly minor, like another child making a sound, triggered the child's stress response to a tipping point where they abruptly reacted.

Children with autism may not outwardly demonstrate any perceived emotion, but internally they may be registering a severe level of emotional distress. Physiological measures allow you to visualize the child's reactions to their environment from the inside out and are thus invaluable for measuring the child's internal stress response during interactions that can occur with parents, peers, staff, and the surrounding environment. We have also found that they are particularly helpful and informative for children with autism who have unusual responses to the environment, limited verbal skills, or may not demonstrate the typical facial and body language cues that clearly show frustration or distress. Understanding the child's state of stress or calmness is helpful if you're teaching because it can guide your interactions.

For example, for the children in our research program we can successfully determine when to present new information that demands attention and concentration based on the child's level of calmness. We know when the child is in a readiness state to learn, which may not be a state without any stress as a little stress is positive for learning as it summons attention. The technology that we use has been particularly helpful after a child experiences a negative behavior. We are beginning to predict with much more accuracy when we believe that the child has calmed down enough in order to return to the lesson at hand. Without insight into the child's internal stress state, teachers and clinicians often put demands on them too soon after a behavior occurred and before the child was ready to reengage simply because they appeared outwardly calm.

Sara Jane Webb, researcher at the Seattle Children's Hospital, and other colleagues in the field of autism have been mounting evidence that physiological measures could help with interventions and could be very useful and informative during screenings and evaluations of children who have autism (Schoen *et al.* 2008; Webb *et al.* 2011). We have used physiological measures and recorded observations to measure the co-regulation that occurs between staff and the child, and child to child. The results have been very illuminating as we seen that there are children in the class who become very anxious when their peers become upset, and like a cascade, when one child becomes stressed and upset, the entire class can become stressed, including the staff. We have had to rethink what we thought was causing some of the symptoms of autism for some children, which has led to new and different interventions.

The technology needed for routine physiological monitoring is becoming more available to parents and to others supporting children with autism in the general public. An ideal scenario and goal for the future would be for a child to be able to wear a physiological sensor when going out to dinner with their family. In this scenario, the parents will have a cell phone that is synchronized with the sensor the child is wearing. If the child begins to sense that the restaurant is over-stimulating and to experience increased stress levels, the parent's cell phone vibrates to signal that they should take the child out of the restaurant. They can then calm down using a de-stressing technique, which will help to prevent a potential public scene.

This type of monitoring is especially powerful for the child who has difficulty communicating or who isn't aware of or in control of their internal stress response. Ultimately, the child could be taught to self-regulate by becoming more aware of their emotions, thus becoming more capable of employing self-calming techniques. There are many other ways that new technologies can lend insights and support in helping children and families. One of our young adults enrolled in a yoga class so that he could learn to deep breathe when he felt himself becoming upset. He is part of our new staff training and orientation program, and has begun to teach new staff at The Center about the need to take deep breaths while working if feeling stressed. The young adult had a history of very aggressive behaviors, but has now learned to self-regulate after becoming aware of his internal stress state. He has enrolled in the gym, is eating a wholefoods diet, and is practicing yoga breaths for relaxation.

The use of technology has helped us rethink why behaviors occur and has been an inspiration in writing this book and in looking deeper at the primary causes of behaviors. The technology is not the answer to solving behaviors, but it is the catalyst for asking more questions. The goal in our program is to gather basic physiological and audio/video data on children and then integrate that information with other important factors that are known to affect stress levels and functioning such as the amount and quality of sleep, bowel functioning, food quality and quantity, seizures, medications, and other health and personally relevant data. All the data is analyzed together in order to get a complete sense of how the child is functioning and what support personnel for children with autism can do to help reduce stress. You don't need technology to begin to help your child. This book will teach you basic strategies that you can use today in your home and in the school or work environment.

INCONSISTENT RESPONSES TO STRESS

We have seen children with autism who exhibit higher than normal and often prolonged reactions to certain individual stressors in the social and physical environments. This phenomenon has been confirmed in many published scientific studies (Tomanik, Harris and Hawkins 2004; Corbett and Simon 2013). These responses or reactions can be different from day to day, and are often influenced or made worse by other biological problems. These findings are consistent with children who have undergone similar analysis in other programs. Prior to these insights and without the many new scientific studies, stressors leading to a behavior were essentially invisible to the parent or behavior analyst. In many behavioral episodes the antecedent or trigger for the behavior cannot be directly correlated to or can be miscorrelated to the behavior—at least until now. This is important because you need to understand why a child is exhibiting a behavior if your treatment is to be successful. For example, if you are suffering with pain from an infected tooth, you may take an aspirin to reduce the pain, but it will not cure the root cause of the pain—an infected tooth. The same logic holds true for a child with autism.

For example, a child with autism may flip over a table in response to particular noise in the environment that is causing them undue stress. If a clinician develops a behavior plan to treat the behavior by having the child pick up the table five times after they flip the table over, a form of over-correction, the problem causing the stress is still not addressed. Likewise, the teacher may decide to bolt the table down so that the table can't flip over, but again the stress on the child still exists and will most likely be exhibited in another way.

Some of the children we observe have what appear to be inconsistencies in their responses. For example, one day a humming noise in the environment may upset the child so much so that they hit another child or may engage in self-abusive behavior like hitting their head on the floor or wall; then on another day, that same humming noise may not affect the child at all. This is confusing at best to the behavior analyst who is looking for the definitive cause of the behavior through observational data.

As is turns out, the child's physiological state—state of stress in the body—can be more heightened from one day to the next, so that on some days they may be in more of an agitated state right from the start than they are on other days. The child is then less tolerant of things like extraneous noises or other interfering problems encountered during the typical day. Observers often miss this subtle nuance, as the degree of behavioral response can be different day to day and sometimes hour to hour. Staff or family members will often assume that there are concrete, externally motivated and immediate antecedents or reasons for poor or unusual behavior, such as dropping to the ground, running away, or seeking attention through screaming or hitting. The professionals then devise behavioral plans to remediate these problems based on what they can see from a restricted, outside, observational vantage point.

Behavior problems seen in children with autism may be caused or affected by things that are not readily observable such as pain, lack of sleep, poor food quality or quantity, abnormal bowel elimination patterns, lack of structure, lack of communication, or a combination of all those and other factors affecting the biological system of the child. There is any number of reasons that a child may exhibit signs of stress or maladaptive behavior, but usually there is something biological or environmental triggering the stress or "fight or flight" response that needs deeper understanding and more than just a real-time human observation. As noted in the study by Harvard University, the response to the complexity in autism needs to be multifaceted and multidisciplinary from the medical perspective.

Just recently an article appeared in the New York Times, "Losing the home he knows" (February 1, 2015), which cited a parent of an individual with autism who sued a program because the program failed to properly diagnose and treat their child's abscessed tooth. Instead the psychiatrist prescribed antipsychotic drugs for the self-injurious behaviors. The family was awarded $625,000 for pain and suffering. Solely because the individual was nonverbal and couldn't tell anyone of his extreme pain, no one thought his behaviors could be linked to pain. This article is an example of a scenario that is injurious for all parties. No one wins when a child suffers.

STRESS

A natural part of a child's development is to experience what has been termed a "stress response." Activation of the stress response is a biological function. It's a protective response that each of us possesses and actually needs to survive. The physical response of stress in the body is set in motion by a perceived threat from one of our senses. Once a threat is perceived, a series of chemical responses occur in the body. The threat does not need to be just physical; it can be psychological, environmental, or emotional.

It is important for us to know how stress is caused if we want to help our children and ourselves. Children with autism typically experience continuous stress as they try to understand the social, emotional, and the temporal complexity of the world around them (Bergland 2014). Here is an example and basic explanation of what happens when we perceive threat:

Picture a child who has autism playing with his toy cars, lining them up, one by one, row by row. He is contented and outwardly relaxed enough to repeat this scenario for hours, seemingly oblivious to what is going on around him.

Then a threat appears. Another child enters the room and wants to join in the play. The child with autism immediately becomes observably anxious. His pace and breath quickens and his hands begin to tremor. He may physically turn away or turn to protect his toy cars. He may even reach out and push the other child if he gets too close. He is threatened by the intrusion into his world of "autistic aloneness" as Leo Kanner describes.

Once this assumed threat is perceived, the internal mechanisms of the child go on high alert. The energy in our brain and body needed for long-term survival is immediately shifted to the short-term problem. In order to protect the body, muscles will need energy to be activated, and the lungs will need more oxygen. The pain response will be blunted and digestion will need to be interrupted—there is no time for food when your life is under threat. The body almost immediately reprioritizes all its functions for survival.

Internally there are whole systems and organs of the body that begin to respond immediately and simultaneously to a perceived threat with the sole purpose of protecting the body. The next few sections will explain some of those primal systems and their actions on the brain and body. These are the systems that affect children with autism the most, and if activated too frequently or for sustained periods of time can cause serious long term health problems. Much of our research and our treatment techniques are aimed at reducing the stress affect to not only help the children learn, but to secure their future from a health perspective.

Adrenaline and cortisol

The adrenal gland sits on top of the kidneys. When activated by a perceived threat, this gland excretes chemicals called epinephrine (adrenaline) and cortisol. The adrenaline increases the heart rate, which sends blood to the muscles and the major organs. The bronchial tubes dilate and the lungs fill with oxygen and extra oxygen is sent to the brain. Hair on the body actually stands up on end as blood vessels constrict ensuring that there is less blood if you were to sustain an injury. The adrenaline also works to release stored glucose, the body's energy.

Made from cholesterol, cortisol, the body's second major stress hormone, is extremely helpful in preparing the body and brain to flee or fight. It works immediately to begin to restore the energy depleted by the adrenaline release. However, cortisol is also responsible for brain destruction if it is not immobilized by other body and brain counter calming chemicals. Cortisol also enhances the storage of energy in the form of fat—particularly the fat seen around the abdomen. In other words, cortisol can contribute to unhealthy weight gain. It can deplete the body of certain proteins and minerals needed for healthy bone growth. Too much cortisol depresses the immune system. However, just enough cortisol allows the body to wake up and attend just after resting, and to recover from an infection. It's a delicate balance.

Chronic stress causing increased activation of cortisol in the body and brain can be a major problem. Particularly susceptible to damage from cortisol is the hippocampus in the brain. The hippocampus is important because it is critical for learning and memory. The renowned brain researcher, Robert Sapolsky (1998), has demonstrated that sustained stress or chronic stress can permanently damage the hippocampus, negatively affecting learning and memory. This is one of the primary health problems that results from long-term stress activation.

Activation of the stress response by a real or a perceived threat also diverts glucose from the brain. Glucose is the brain's food. This causes further problems in the brain's hippocampus, as it requires glucose for energy. Thus, learning and memory are negatively affected.

Children with autism already experience difficulty in the learning environment because of problems with communication and social skills. They do not need added damage to the hippocampus or other primary brain structures because of sustained stress exposure. As a provider of programs for children with autism, careful attention must be paid to each child and their environments to ensure they feel safe and secure, and know what is expected of them to prevent the stress response. There are more systems that go into alert or "fight or flight" mode when stressed including the autonomic nervous system.

The autonomic nervous system

As explained in the previous section, stress impacts a person biologically, as well as psychologically. For children with autism, this can be particularly dangerous over time. In this section, you will learn about the role of the autonomic nervous system (ANS) and its relationship to children with autism. The more equipped you are with both psychological and biological information, the better able you will be to help your child live a healthy, productive life.

When a person experiences stress their ANS goes into high gear. This occurs to all of us, regardless of our age and genetic makeup. This complex system automatically regulates metabolism, which keeps the body in balance. It controls functions like respiration and heart rate, digestion, immune and sexual functions, perspiration, pupillary dilation, urination, and swallowing.

Whether under real or perceived stress conditions, the ANS essentially tells the body to decrease digestion, immune, urine, and sexual functioning, while simultaneously telling it to increase breathing, heart rate, perspiration, and pupil dilation. These messages prepare the body for a fight or flight response to defeat the enemy or to get away. In other words, the body is preparing itself to go into battle to defeat the enemy or to get away as quickly as possible. Additionally, the adrenaline that is released from the adrenal gland causes a rapid release of glucose and fatty acids into the bloodstream, causing your senses to become keener and less sensitive to pain, and your muscles to become activated. When all of this occurs together, you are in metabolic overdrive— at least for the moment until the perceived threat is gone and the calming part of the ANS, the parasympathetic nervous system (PSNS), responds with a counter effect—the "rest and digest" effect (Fox 1996).

Stress, believe it or not, allows us to survive. A small amount of daily stress gives us the energy we need to tackle each day, and the stress response can save our life if we are in real danger. However, as much as our brains have evolved over thousands of years, the energy release during the stress response is still that of the very primitive, intense and swift response essentially used to escape the jaws of the saber tooth tiger.

Picture yourself driving down the road late for an important appointment. A car pulls out of a side road and cuts you off. As if that's not enough to get your blood boiling, the car then slows down to 20 mph in a 40 mph zone, and you can't pass the car. Out of sheer frustration you begin to blow your horn. The driver continues at a snail's pace. You can feel the frustration in your body growing. You have no recourse other than breaking the law. This is the point at which road rage can occur for some who are at their tipping point. The brain can simply snap into a rage. However, the brain doesn't really just snap. The pressure is cumulative. It builds over time with repeated stress exposures and no relief. The reasonable response would be to self-calm or self-regulate by perhaps breathing deeply or diverting your attention to something else. In this scenario, your body has just experienced the stress system in action. Think about it—the society in which we live in has become so stressful, we now have a term like road rage to describe this stress response. As people living in modern society, we are at such heightened states of mind that it only takes a little push to tip us over the edge.

The experience you felt in this scenario is the same as the cave men experienced in response to stress. The body system became flooded with a series of chemical and biological reactions meant to help you survive. This is a lifesaving response if you indeed need lifesaving, but it can also be detrimental to your health if you can't shut the system down or regulate it.

Unfortunately and most importantly, the body cannot survive this intense response if it's chronic. If the response does not subside long enough for the body to go back to a dynamic equilibrium state of rest, it will eventually suffer all the negative consequences of stress. A prolonged or high frequency stress response over time will result in a cascade of poor health and medical problems. Therein lies the problem of chronic stress. Calvin's story is an example of a teenage boy who came to live in our residential program because he was out of control in his home environment and his parents and teachers couldn't help him any more.

CALVIN'S STORY

Calvin was admitted into our school program after being moved out of his home at age 15 because of his extreme self-injurious and harmful aggressive behaviors that seemingly were unprovoked much of the time. He was nonverbal and cried often; doctors could find nothing wrong with him. He had a very poor diet high in processed foods and sugar, was overweight, and didn't sleep well. According to his mother, Calvin was not happy. He wasn't always like this, but over time his problems became much worse. She was heartbroken for him and her family. It was evident that Calvin was regressing.

He was enrolled in our research program to better understand the origins of his behaviors. After several months, it was discovered that Calvin had an extreme sensitivity to certain noises, a sensitivity that was affected by his gastrointestinal functioning and his sleep pattern. By using the physiological stress monitoring system, the team at The Center could visualize when Calvin was externally and internally stressed. All the information that was being collected about the food he was eating, how he was sleeping, how his stomach and digestive system were functioning, and how he was able to function during the day was integrated and examined on a daily basis. As it turned out, he was more irritable on days when he was constipated and not sleeping well. This pattern of behavior was not evident until all the data could be visualized together within an integrated system.

The story for Calvin has a very happy ending. Medical and clinical interventions were initiated to address his gastrointestinal and sleep problems. Calvin is now thriving and experiences very few self-injurious or aggressive behaviors. His mother describes Calvin as being happy and smiling every time she sees him. All she has ever wanted was for Calvin to be happy, and now he is. The family can travel for five hours in a car together, and have dinner in new restaurants, activities that were not possible before. Calvin's world has opened up and learning has once again become possible.

WHY WE NEED TO ADDRESS STRESS IN CHILDREN WITH AUTISM

Many of the behaviors seen in a child with autism are often described as happening "out of the blue" by clinicians and parents; however, this is inaccurate. These behaviors do not come from out of nowhere, nor do they happen simply because that the child does not want to participate in what's going on around them. Chronic stress, caused by environmental, cellular-biological, psychological, or emotional factors, is a major culprit in how children with autism respond to circumstances in their surroundings on a day-to-day, minute-by-minute basis. In order to develop the right interventions at the right time for the child, it is critically important to understand the particular cause(s) of stress.

How can we begin to teach children with autism if they are experiencing chronic stress and the associated problems that are brought on by chronic stress? It's quite plausible that many of the maladaptive responses, like aggressive or self-injurious behaviors, seen in children with autism can be a direct result of the wear and tear on their bodies and brains due to chronic stress. Stress may come from many sources such as an unpredictable event, a sudden change in a routine, lack of focused attention, a new or challenging social event, toxins in the environment affecting the body, or an internal response to pain or persistent discomfort. Stress is made worse when it builds up over time from one situation to the next.

As expressed in their research, Groden and colleagues (Groden *et al*. 1994) have found that many of the behaviors in autism are actually related to stress conditions, which precipitate maladaptive behaviors such as aggression, self-abuse, tantrums, and property destruction (Prior and Ozonoff 1998). At The Center, we are seeing this very same phenomenon—many of the behaviors are precipitated by a rise in the internal stress state, which may or may not be obvious to the observer, but are being recorded in real time by their electrodermal activity (EDA). The stress states can be triggered by any number of external events, but typically the child is primed by some internal biological problem that exacerbates the reaction to the external event. In Calvin's case, he had very difficult days when he wasn't sleeping well and when his bowels were irregular. His stress level elevated much more quickly in response to events on these days than it did on days when he was feeling better.

The idea of stress being elevated on days that we aren't feeling well shouldn't come as a surprise to us. Most likely on days when you experience lack of sleep or pain, such as from a head or toothache, you are less tolerant of those around you. This response is compounded if those around you are making demands on you.

About a month ago, I experienced my first sinus infection. I awoke in the morning and immediately was faced with a severe splitting headache that started in my right cheek and traveled right up though my nose, eyes, and forehead. My husband jokingly told me that I looked awful. I did look awful, and I felt awful. But instead of agreeing, I ended up yelling at him for his insensitive comment. I was in such pain that I had no tolerance for his humor. Had he told me the day before that I looked awful, I would have probably just laughed.

After taking two aspirin, I went to work. Things went further downhill from there. The phone calls started. My schedule was double booked, and everyone seemed to need something immediately. I ended up having to walk out of my office before I screamed. My head was ready to explode, and so was I. Luckily, I had the wherewithal to go my doctor's office. Problem solved—I found out I had an acute sinus infection and was put on an antibiotic. In 48 hours, I was as good as new. I was feeling better, but more importantly for those around me, my stress was completely relieved. I am not suggesting that all behaviors seen in children with autism arise out of acute illnesses; what I am suggesting is that if there are chronic underlying conditions from unresolved biological problems or chronic stress, the tolerance that a child has for life's daily demands will be greatly diminished.

Unfortunately for children with more complex forms of autism, daily stress can be chronic. Many programs for children with autism unfortunately and often unknowingly promote stress conditions, as threat and reward are commonly practiced as a basis of control over the child while other health problems are ignored. Processed foods with high amounts of sugar content are often given as rewards for correct responses or good behavior. Over time these rewards equate to added stress and inflammation in the body resulting in poor behavior. The initial results in these programs might be promising in that the child may respond correctly for a cookie, but from an overall health perspective these approaches can be harmful.

It's no secret that chronically stressed brains cannot learn. The brain begins to lose its ability to retain and learn new information under chronic stress and threat conditions, especially in the area of the brain called the hippocampus. Bauman and Kemper (2005) have found that some individuals with autism have decreased and more densely packed neurons in the hippocampus. The potentially damaging hormone, cortisol, which is excreted into the blood, has been found to be more prolonged and at higher levels in children with autism (Spratt *et al.* 2012). There are myriad problems caused by chronic stress affecting health in many children with autism. These problems are evidenced in the child and often seen as:

* gastrointestinal and bowel problems

* eczema and other skin problems

* sleep problems

* obesity and/or pre-diabetic, or underweight

* severe anxiety

* extreme irritability often resulting in maladaptive behaviors.

Parents have revealed other health problems in their children with autism. Unfortunately, according to information we have gathered from our parents and as cited in other studies, some physicians and professionals may attribute health problems as being part of autism—ones that often go untreated (Spratt *et al.* 2012). Science and medical professionals know with certainty what happens to a body that suffers years of chronic stress without proper treatment and the outlook is not good. Medical problems in autism need to be treated.

Professionals in the field are just beginning to understand the relationship between stress and autism, but it's been clinically acknowledged since Dr. Leo Kanner's (1943) first description of autism. Children with autism are under tremendous stress on a daily basis from what they perceive as threat conditions. In recognition of the need to find ways to reduce stress conditions on the child, four essential elements have been outlined, which when regulated effectively should result in stress reduction and improved health, vitality and functioning of the child.

Stress—it's not just the child's problem

Moms, dads, sisters, brothers, and grandparents this paragraph is for you. Co-regulation of emotions occurs between children with autism and others in their environment. When children get upset or stressed, others in the environment can also experience emotional stress. The converse is also true. When adults experience stress, this response can cause a similar reaction for the child. If the child is in a larger group and is stressed, the total stress level for the group rises as well. Learning about stress and learning to regulate and decrease your stress is the first step in helping your child regulate and decrease their stress. No one wins when everyone is stressed. Regulating the stress response is not always easy and it takes time, but it's a necessity. Strategies for decreasing stress are expressed in the core chapters of this book.

THE FIRST STEP TOWARD DECREASING STRESS

The first step toward decreasing stress is becoming aware of the feeling of being stressed and understanding what might be causing the stress. Parents will often say that they do not have time to think about themselves and their stress, or they say that they are always stressed and that's just the way it is. Many children with autism and their parents are following a trajectory similar to those suffering from health problems brought on by chronic anxiety and stress. I'm not suggesting that the core symptoms of autism arise out of the consequence of stress; more likely they are major contributors to chronic stress and anxiety. I am suggesting that if the child's health problems are not addressed and stress is not reduced, the child will follow a trajectory similar to those who have chronic disease, which indisputably equates to a shorter and decreased quality of life. The same holds true for parents of children with autism.

Because of the problems seen in the children who we evaluate, we have assembled a team of clinicians and researchers to help us discern which interventions, methods, and program designs work best, and positively affect the long term health and development of children with autism. Helping a child with autism heal is not a quick fix. It's a lifestyle approach with essential components outlined in a guiding framework, which will be detailed in the next set of chapters.

ASSEMBLING YOUR TEAM

You need help when raising a child with complex autism. Don't be shy about reaching out for help. Even if you only have one lifeline, you are off to a really good start. As a parent or a person who is supporting a child with autism, you may want to assemble your own team to help. Below are short descriptors of the team members and their roles. You can be flexible in assembling your team. The most important point is that they should support you and your child.

* an advocate—someone who isn't afraid to speak and help you in meetings and in getting the right services for your child and who can take notes or remind you of what you want to say

* an organizer—someone who loves to make lists and schedules, and probably loves the Container store—the store that just sells containers; they can help you develop the strategies and schedules needed to externally organize your child

* a chef—someone who knows about nutrition and can cook healthy meals with fresh whole foods and provide simple cooking and eating lessons and menus

* a Zen friend—someone who is unflappable in the face of crisis, is very calm and health conscious and can help you relax and provide strategies to help your child relax

* a child sitter—someone who knows about autism, has patience, and likes children

* a balancer—a good listener who doesn't judge.

The advocate

There are many valuable resources that can help you find team members such as Autism Speaks,[1] which consists of a large number of parents, family members, and scientists who provide a wealth of online information and resources about autism. These resources are all meant to help parents and caregivers of children with autism. When you visit this site, click on "Resources Guide," which will take you to a map of your state. Just scroll down to the Advocacy section, and you should find many valuable resources with some states having more than others. If you're not finding what you want, search online for "advocacy services for child with in autism in My Town, USA." On this site, you will find many government funded, free resources and grant sponsored resources that are not listed on the Autism Speaks site. You may also want to reach out to your local community or school, which will often have support groups for parents or information about support groups. Your child's pediatrician should be a good source of information, as pediatricians are seeing an increased number of children in their practices and have access to wealth of updated information.

The organizer

Parents are often great at helping other parents. I have seen parents who are talented chefs get other parents together to host a

---

1   www.autismspeaks.org

"healthy cooking with the kids" Saturday activity. It's educational, organized, functional, and fun! Each parent can volunteer to be one of the team leaders depending on their area of interest or talent. For example, the "organized parent" can host a "let's get organized for school party." This can be a day where children and parents come together and make schedules and create and label bins to keep their work in order. Getting organized is really important but often difficult as parents face minute-to-minute demands as they are trying to care for their child. You can look online for "how do busy parents stay organized?" and you will find scores of organizational tips, strategies, and programs, many of which are online and free, and well as services for hire that will help you organize and declutter. Doing this with other parents is a great way to connect, get work done, and have children interact with each other. There are also many great teachers who are willing to help with strategies and tips on helping children interact during these gatherings.

The chef

If you're not a chef, and most of us aren't, do not fret. I have included some really easy and practical cooking tips, lessons, and recipes in the chapter on eating and nutrition. However, if you need assistance with cooking, you may find resources that are free through your local college or high school. Many of these students are required to do community service, and teaching parents of children with autism how to prepare whole foods would be a very worthy endeavor. Your child or children can even join in on the fun. There is also a great online site where you'll find terrific videos like Bobby Flay's "Healthy Picks... Plan, Shop, Eat,"[2] as well as many other free online videos featuring children that may attract your child to watch, learn, and enjoy cooking! Watch for

2   www.foodnetwork.com

upcoming videos on The Center for Discovery website with Master Chef Cesare Casella on cooking for health.[3]

The Zen

Your Zen friend, if you have one, is probably someone who would be happy to help. By virtue of their calm nature, they may be an important person in your pursuit for a less stressful existence. Whether or not you find a Zen friend, it will behove you to find methods for remaining calm in the face of a crisis and through mounting, daily stress. Yoga, as discussed in the chapter on emotional regulation, can be a wonderful strategy to help you and your family to keep calm and carry on. Before you dismiss the thought as impossible for your child, take a look at the Kripalu website.[4] Kripalu is a wonderful Center for Yoga and Health in the Berkshires of Western Massachusetts, and their online shop offers many instructional DVDs to bring yoga into your home, several of which are made for children and with children. They can be extremely motivating and instructional for a child with autism. If you want to visit Kripalu, they offer family programs that incorporate healthy eating and yoga practice, all while being immersed in the natural beauty of the Berkshires. You can embrace the four essential components in this book while on a family vacation. If it's not in your budget, call Kripalu as they offer scholarships in some cases. You should also reach out to your local yoga instructors, of which there are usually many, who may volunteer their time to help especially if they have an interest in children with autism.

The sitter

It is well documented fact that raising a child with autism is more expensive than raising a neurotypical child and discretionary

3   www.thecenterfordiscovery.org
4   https://shop.kripalu.org

spending is often limited as a result (Lavelle *et al.* 2014). If you don't have money to hire a sitter or friends or family available to help out, there are resources available to you. Often times there are family support grants that you can access through government or non-government organizations. Autism Speaks and other similar organizations may be able to help. Grants may be available in the form of vouchers, ranging from $400–$1000 per family per year. If your area doesn't offer these resources, I suggest that you reach out to your local high school or college, as they typically have mandatory community service programs, and/or students enrolled in psychology and education programs who may have an interest in spending time with children with autism. Often times student interns or those doing community service are willing to support you for free or more cheaply than an average sitter.

The balancer

A balancer is someone who will listen to your frustrations, hopes, and dreams without judging. They should be someone you trust and can confide in. If you don't have a friend or family member who you consider a balancer, then seek out the support of a clergy person, therapist, or someone who is trained to listen to and support those who are struggling or in crisis. You may not need this person all the time, but it's good to have someone you trust in your back pocket.

Parents can also work with other parents to pool their resources and hire the team member that they might be missing. The point is that you should not ever feel alone. You can be appreciated in a team format for whatever talent you may have—and you only need one talent to contribute!

A WORD ABOUT CONSISTENCY

Consistent ways of interacting and stability amongst team members supporting a child with autism are critical. Children with autism thrive on consistency—that is, having routines and knowing what is expected with well-planned change. Being part of a team is more of an art form than a step by step process. It requires dynamic give and take and relentless commitment from everyone. The team should have a designated leader who is able to keep the ball rolling and is motivating with a sense of humor. Humor is really important because the work of the team can be stressful, and stress can interfere with functioning. Humor keeps things lighthearted.

I suggest rotating team members into the leadership position to keep things fresh and energized. Your team should decide on one way of best communicating with each other such as text message, group email, or journaling by sharing entries. The use of group email tends to work best for everyday communication. It only takes one email to reach everyone, and team members can review and respond to communications at their leisure. Text messaging should be reserved for the very important communications. It's helpful if the team meets at least once per month and decides what the most important issues are that need to be communicated. The important issues are usually ones that are interfering with daily functioning, such as a behavior that the child may be experiencing, a medical problem that requires monitoring, or a significant problem in a particular area in school. A clear plan of action that focuses on solutions should be decided upon, and each team member should be clear about where they fit in with supporting the child. The leader guides the team to ensure everyone stays focused and responsive.

SUMMARY

My hope is that you are well on your way toward seeing autism as more than its core symptoms as described in the DSM 5. I encourage you to use your intuition and observation when thinking about your child—be your own diagnostician to discover what the greatest sources of stress are for your child and for yourself. Assemble your team and work with the professionals who are supporting and educating your child.

In the next set of chapters, you will discover the key elements that can be regulated on a day-to-day basis to begin to help reduce stress and improve functioning for your child. These four chapters are meant to be put into action.

PART 2

Chapter 4

ENVIRONMENTAL REGULATION

The environment is the first of the four components that can be regulated in order to help your child function better. The essential elements of the environment include the physical, temporal, and social components. In this chapter, you will learn ways to adjust or change the environment to provide the best outcome for your child.

However, before looking at emotional regulation in detail I want to briefly discuss the concept of regulation.

A WORD ABOUT REGULATING

Now that you have read the first set of chapters, you are ready to begin to help your child. Before you start, I'd like to share a story about how and why I chose to use the framework of regulating, and what regulating means.

My choice begins with my grandfather, Norbert, who was Chief Engineer for McAllister Tug Boats in New York City. I share this story because it was during my trips to the engine room with my grandfather that I learned about the importance of knowing how to regulate an engine to keep the tug boat functioning at peak performance. The principle of regulating an engine is the same principle used in thinking about regulating our body's systems to improve functioning.

I distinctly recall my grandfather talking about the importance of the regulators, which essentially controlled the operations of the motors and ultimately the fate of the tug and its crew. The regulators managed and maintained a range of preset values that kept the motor running at optimal levels. The main regulator, the brain of the engine, was responsible for maintaining an optimum engine speed so that the tug could push or pull the massive barges without losing its momentum and power. That meant that at certain times the engine automatically called on and regulated different parts of the system to increase power or decrease power in a highly coordinated way. Key regulators in the engine room controlled a set of key functions, and all had to work in harmony to maintain peak functioning.

I've often thought about these regulators from a conceptual framework, that is, how important regulating is to human performance and functioning. What is it that regulates us, preventing us from just going haywire or from losing energy? What keeps us functioning at our optimum peaks? What do we need to do to muster up just the right amount of energy to attend and likewise what do we need to turn down energy to relax or sleep? And, most importantly, how can we control these regulating systems?

As it turns out, our body and brain are dynamic systems changing and continuously adjusting and regulating in response to our own experiences. We have internal regulators constantly adjusting to our experiences. And, as chief engineers of our bodies and brains, we have certain control over these regulators. So it stands to reason that if we become conscious of what's important to regulate for optimizing functioning, then we can actively affect change. That's what this book is about—learning to actively and consciously regulate our experiences and affect change.

You can learn to dial up or dial down the key components to functioning that have been identified as explained in the next set of chapters. For example, sometimes you may need to dial down (calm) the excitement of the environment or dial up (increase) energy in order to help your child to focus; or you may need to dial up nutrition (better quality food) and dial down energy (relaxation) in order to help your child sleep at night. Once you understand what you can regulate, you will be on your way toward making life more positive for your child.

It's important to remember that each child and each family are individuals, so how you implement the essentials of this framework and to what extent is up to you; what's important to understand is that each of the essential components plays an important role in combating stress and promoting health.

Parents who have experienced this framework report that their children are happier and are able to interact and function better in their homes with their families and in the community. For me, that's the best indicator of all.

THE GOAL OF THIS BOOK

This book aims to help the whole family. By consciously integrating the components of this framework into daily life, the whole family can begin to see the positive outcomes expected through this model. The four essential components, environment, emotional-self, eating and nutrition, and energy are not mystical, nor are they highly complex. They are well documented in the literature and practical such that you can begin to implement them now.

Take a moment to think about how much you already know about raising or supporting a child with autism from a health perspective. If you are a parent, you have amassed a tremendous amount of knowledge that can be applied to this model.

Now on a scale of one through seven, rate yourself on how much you think you already know about stress on your child. How much do you know about implementing strategies to help reduce stress and to foster an atmosphere of growth in the key areas noted below? After each chapter, you can rate your knowledge again and hopefully with each page that you read, you learn something new.

Scoring a one means you really know very little about the essential components outlined in the first section of this book; scoring a seven means that you are very well versed about the components and are staying up to date about new findings; scoring a four means you are somewhere in the middle, but you're on your way toward a healthier future. Regardless of how well versed you are, this book offers a new way of thinking about autism, along with new methods for caring for a child with autism. So, the scale of 1–7 is just a starting point. The important part is the journey that begins in reading this book and putting the information gleaned into action in your life.

Reflecting on my own journey in teaching children with complex problems, I would score myself very low on all elements in the beginning years of my experience. My initial thoughts, not unlike many new professionals in the field, were that children with autism had learning and problems with brain functioning, which led to severe behaviors that made life really challenging. I also thought that by using good teaching and behavioral methodologies, I could make tremendous strides in helping my students learn. That turned out not to be the case, which is how I came to realize that I needed a lot more information from many more sources including the medical and science community in order to really help long term. Three decades later, I'm still not seven on the scale on all accounts, but I am continuing to learn and I'm able to help a lot more children, families, and professionals as a result of my learning.

1	4	7
Little knowledge		Very knowledgeable

Note: What to do I need to do to get closer to a seven?

The first section below describes the physical environment and includes the built and natural environments; the second is the temporal environment having to do with routines and timing of activities and events; and the third section describes the components of the social environment where the child learns to feel safe and secure in the presence of others and during interactions with others.

In his observations of children with autism, Kanner (1943) found that these three components of the environment were problematic. He noted that children with autism were greatly affected by and became highly anxious in situations that had to do with the physical space, time, activities, and people in the environment. He noted that *sameness* and routine kept the child calm and in control and likewise intrusions and unpredictability made the child highly anxious and stressed.

Today, we observe the same indicators in our observations of children with all levels of autism. All three of these dimensions of the environment affect the internal state of the child, and can either promote a calming and pleasant effect or induce a stress response. There are children we work with who can become distressed when their routines are changed or when they need to transition from one activity to another. How we regulate the environmental components can either help or hinder a child's response. The first step is simply becoming aware of these components.

Remember the little boy who was lining up his cars in the chapter on stress? He was content and stress free until his social environment changed and another child intruded on his space. With the shift in environment, he was overcome by the reactionary stress response. There are actions that could have been taken in this scenario to prevent the debilitating stress response experienced by this little boy.

Instructors could have implemented a time-based schedule designed to prepare the boy ahead of time that another child would be entering his environment. Then he could have practiced this interaction using a specifically designed social story presented in a non-threatening environment. He could have practiced this interaction until he became accustomed to it and the stress response was diminished. Additionally, he could have been taught some techniques for self-calming like deep breathing with progressive muscle relaxation if he felt himself becoming anxious.

Environments and their thoughtful design are critical to a child with autism as they offer the child conscious and unconscious cues about expectations for what should happen in a space (Lackney 2003; Shabha 2006). When expectations for how to act or behave in the environment are made clear to the child and the child is comfortable, the interaction is typically positive and does not evoke a stress response. Conversely, if the child is confused by the environmental expectations or finds the environment overwhelming and unpredictable, the response may not be a positive one. You can help to regulate your child's environment in order to help them achieve maximum behavioral success.

THE PHYSICAL ENVIRONMENT

Children with autism are always on guard, every moment, trying to figure out what is expected of them. As a result, they experience fatigue and often and with more intensity then typically developing children. They require more energy to function and thus more rest to restore their systems. A majority of children with autism also have hypersensitivities and heightened senses that affect their ability to attend to activities and to learn (Grandin 1995; Freed and Parsons 1997). Remember, when you're actively in stress mode, your senses are heightened. For these reasons, the first step when designing or locating a space in the environment for learning or play, is to identify the unique needs and strengths of the child.

If you are a parent, you probably know instinctively what environments your child thrives in and on the other hand, which types of environments they struggle with. Whether it's a classroom at school or a room in your home, it is important to conduct an assessment of the indoor space. Begin with the layout of the built environment. Homes are usually smaller and simpler in design, which is good because it is easier to figure out the layout. Make a list of the environments that your child seems to do well in and conversely those that they may not do well in. For example, your child may not like environments that have a certain noise or high ceilings that echo with sound. Share this list with your child's school personnel and other key people who may be interacting with your child. You know your child the best, and this information is critical in creating environments that your will child will thrive in.

If the child with autism feels safe and secure in the environment, there is less of a chance that their stress response will be heightened. Use of color, furniture, furniture arrangement, lighting, air exchange, sound/acoustics, and room dimensions are all important features to consider in the built environments. Aesthetics and the physical design and materials in the physical environment can help. Temple Grandin helped us design the homes for children who live in our residential program. She suggested colors that were muted southwestern colors, and that we create smaller spaces in the environment for the child to retreat to. We also used wood on the floors to absorb sound and create a softer feel to the environment. Additionally, there were many windows to allow lots of natural light and views of nature, and good cross ventilation.

What is most important for the child in the home is that they have a place that feels safe where they can retreat to if there is a situation that is overwhelming or if they are exhausted from the demands of the day. A safe space should be designated for the child that is quiet and comfortable perhaps with a hanging swing, a large ball to lay and bounce on, or a rocking chair. The space should also have a door to close to dampen sound and visual noise that can be overwhelming. This space may be the child's bedroom or other designated quiet area.

As you conduct your assessment of the child's spaces note the size of the space, the kind of furniture and its arrangement in the space, the sound level, organization, and the colors. It can be easy to acclimatize to spaces that we are most familiar with and miss the very details that children with autism readily see. It can thus be helpful to have someone with fresh eyes and an objective opinion come in and conduct an evaluation. The features of the environment that can influence how well the child performs in the space are discussed below.

The home and school environments

In this section, I discuss steps to take for the physical design in the two most integral environments for a child with autism: the home and school. There is consideration for how these environments affect the child's senses. Some environments facilitate functioning and some hinder functioning and trigger a stress response.

Home environment

The furniture in the home environment should be considered as a factor in helping a child navigate their environment. Furniture offers visual cues and subtle rules about what is expected to happen in the environment. Children with autism thrive when they understand rules and expectations. In the home environment, for example, a bedroom usually contains a bed—the bed signals the child to lie down; this is where sleep happens. The bedroom should be the quietest space for the child. The bathroom and kitchen are typically easier to interpret as there is highly contextual cueing in these environments via the toilet, tub, sink, stove, refrigerator, etc. The child may not be fully proficient in the activities that occur in these environments such as being independent in taking a shower; however, there is a general understanding of what should occur in these spaces. If you use the kitchen table for activities other than eating, you should be clear about what time activities happen. For example, in the morning the kitchen table or counter is most likely just used for eating breakfast; however, after school the kitchen table may be the homework table. You need to make sure that your child understands the multipurpose use of this table.

Because of their tendency toward multipurpose functioning, living rooms, family rooms, and dining rooms can be more complex, similar to a classroom environment. It is in these spaces that furniture becomes multi-use and expectations can change depending on the day, time of day, and activities that take place in the room. It is in these spaces that children with autism have the most difficulty because they may not understand what is expected of them for a particular time.

For example, if you use the dining room table for meals and also use the same table for homework, the child may have difficulty sitting to do their homework if they are expecting to eat dinner. Multipurpose, transitional spaces are not intuitive, and require an understanding of time and being flexible, which children with autism sometimes struggle with. With that in mind, this is where temporal supports and color cueing explicitly designed calendars, schedules, checklists, and sequenced and color-coded picture boards can help the child understand expectations. Temporal (timing/activity) cues should have a consistent place in the environment, such as on a cork or chalk board on the wall. Temporal cues, as described in the next section of this chapter, are explicit, visual, sequential, and typically timed in sequence. Wherever there are spaces that are multipurpose, you need to pay attention. These are the hot spots for stress.

In these hotspot spaces, it is helpful to have a designated, consistent place where the child can sit that is familiar to them and doesn't change. This can help the child feel grounded. Once the child is sitting, you can review the expectations for that particular activity with the child. For example, if the family room is a place to watch TV, play games, talk to others, wait for dinner to be done, and/or listen to music, the child would enter the family room, sit in their designated space, and would be given a verbal and visual cue of what the expectation was for that space, during that time, and for how long it was to occur. As the child becomes more accustomed to their routine, the amount of cueing can be decreased. It helps to conduct a time and motion study for a week or two to discover which spaces in your home are hot spots. It's an easy study that is time based. To do this, document what space your child is in and what they are doing every 15 minutes. Note how many spaces they use, what they use them for, and for how long. If your child simply roams, then you will need to develop an organized schedule to support their learning. Once you are armed with this information, you can begin to help your child understand the expectations that they will need to meet for the each different physical environment.

School environment

The school environment is typically much more complex than the home because it contains many doors, larger floor plans, large and smaller classrooms, and gathering areas with overall acoustics that are often challenging to the child. In addition, almost all space in a school is multipurpose and more often than not, the spaces appear to be cluttered. Expectations are constantly changing in school environments. One day the gym may be used for physical education and the next day for an assembly space. The cafeteria may typically be used for lunch, but can also double as a study hall. Also, the typical classroom can change as it transitions from a reading group lesson with small clusters of chairs and desks to a large group lesson with rows of desks. For some children with autism, this can be confusing if it is not well structured.

It's important to choose a school that is logically designed and if possible, small in size. This equates to a limited number of classrooms with a simple layout, which allows and encourages the child to learn to be independent. For a child with autism, I would avoid the open-school concept where there are no interior walls dividing classroom spaces. If a smaller school is not an option, try limiting the amount of travel and transitions the child has to make during the school day. Less is more for a child with autism; this includes less visually stimulating spaces and as few transitions as possible during the day. Limit the number of changes a child has to adapt to until the child feels safe.

Randall Fielding (2006) has conducted extensive research on school environments. According to his 2006 study, there are a number of thoughtful design aspects that can enhance a sense of belonging in a child. These include:

* individual-scale spaces from a rocking chair or cubby storage space for a pre-kindergartener, to a personal workstation for a middle or senior school student

* family or extended family scale spaces accommodating advisory groups, home units, or project teams of 10, 15 or 20

* small learning communities of 100 to 150 (if the school is very large in numbers of students)

* neighborhoods of two or more small learning communities

* multiple small learning communities and neighborhoods across campus.

Because we have close to 300 children in our school at The Center, we use the neighborhood concept as a way to help the children connect with other children in their environment. They see their neighborhood friends on a daily basis and are engaged in similar activities that surround the neighborhood.

As the child becomes more accustomed to the spaces in the school and more confident, complexity and flexibility can be added. Any changes should be introduced slowly and predictably to allow time to process and accept the changes. You should continually seek to build upon the child's skills and repertoires, but this should be done step by step with careful attention paid to their ability to accept and process change.

Use of learning stations in the classroom is a really great way to help the child stay focused on the activity at hand. You can set up between three and four stations for the child to rotate through during an hour-long lesson. Each activity in each station can have its own micro-schedule and timing for the station. Children with autism thrive in these types of arrangements because they understand what is expected of them. Social skills and peer modeling can be enhanced during these small group-learning stations by using social stories that teach basic social interactions or teaching turn taking and proper social responding.

Children with autism have great difficulty paying attention to what is relevant in situations and spaces, and too many distractions, especially on the walls, can be counterproductive. Walls and spaces should be well organized and clutter free. This does not mean you need to eliminate everything on the wall. I have been in classrooms where teachers have taken everything off their walls in an effort to cut down on distractions. The child's brain needs stimulation and novelty—it thrives on this. We need to find balance in order to help our children thrive.

The use of a ball chair can assist the child who is fidgety. A ball chair is a therapy ball which is placed on a stand to keep it from rolling away. These types of chairs are commercially available and can be found by searching online for "therapy ball chair." Using a ball chair also helps with core body strengthening, which is great for children who have weaker abdominal muscles. If the child becomes over-aroused during the day, the ball can also help modify the arousal state. You should also have a quiet corner available in the classroom. This space should be cosy and may even have noise-cancelling headphones for the child to wear. In classrooms for younger children, I have used a pop-up tent and even large cardboard boxes for a child to retreat into.

In both the home and school environments, it is very important that the child have a place to put their belongings such as books, papers, personal technology, and so on. This space should be highly organized and well labeled in a way that makes sense to the child—alphabetically, color coded, and/or temporally sequenced by activities. If you are not an orderly, organized person, I suggest soliciting help from someone who is. This is important, as an organized approach reduces anxiety and offers a means to success (Hannah 2001). Work with the child to keep the space organized.

There are some children with autism who can become very overwhelmed during transitions from one place to another place. They may try to escape the confusion by running away. Sometimes they run to a place where they feel secure, which is usually a space that offers predictability or one that they are familiar with. Unfortunately, many of these children lack basic safety awareness making these attempts to leave or run away very dangerous.

Children who run without safety awareness

If the child has a propensity for wandering or running that is not safe, it's imperative that the school and homes are equipped with safety features such as door and window alarms, window blocks if needed, and doors that are lockable, especially at night. Some children may also benefit from GPS tracking devices, which are becoming more readily available and reliable with increased battery life. I would recommend a device that has good battery life, and it seems that currently the most reliable systems are the ones that have been trialed in the justice system. These are now being marketed to Life Assist Facilities. Open concept spaces and long linear corridors are not desirable as they can over stimulate and increase the child's desire to run or roam (Gaines, Sancribrian and Lock 2011).

Always make certain that whoever is supporting the child is aware of the wandering or running behavior, and be aware of where the child might want to run to. Places a child run can include their favorite places, like swings, train stations, or water features. These are often where children go when they are compelled to escape. Just as you would practice fire safety with a monthly fire drill procedure, practice what to do if the child escapes with all support personnel.

The most important point is that when there are safety concerns for the child with autism, the entire team including all school administrators and professionals should understand what those concerns are and know what to do in case of an emergency. Every minute counts for a child with autism who could be in danger.

Defining space

A few weeks ago I was giving a lecture to about thirty professionals about space design. I was in the school gym, and there were folding chairs set out for the staff to sit on. I was standing in the front of the room speaking when a very active teenage boy with autism ran into room yelling and bouncing up and down. It was clear that the child was hyper-aroused and ready for gym class. He startled everyone in the lecture, and it was as if we were all frozen in that moment. People were uncertain about what might happen next. Amazingly, the boy looked around, stopped yelling, and darted for the empty seat. He immediately modeled the behavior of the staff, sat appropriately, and listened to the rest of the lecture, which lasted 15 minutes. His behavior was perfect in terms of the expected behavior for the situation.

As I continued my lecture, I was able to use his behavior as an example to support the point that when children are offered cues from their environment, they are then able to understand what is expected of them. When this happens, they can respond without a "fight or flight" response and be in a ready state to learn. This child was cued by the environment and subsequently was able to adapt and be ready to learn.

About an hour later when I was touring the school, I noticed the same child running around a group of 20 or so staff gathered in the hall. He was literally bouncing up in the air at least two feet with each jump. Clearly there were no boundaries or obvious cues as to the expected behavior in the hall. This disorganized state was further exacerbated by the fact that so many staff were gathering in a seemingly haphazard way that appeared to be unusual for the space.

It was clear to me that this was very disorganizing to the child, as he appeared very disruptive and impulsive. He was totally over-aroused. I asked a staff to get a chair for the child since they could not seem to catch him as he was literally bouncing around the group. The staff brought a rolling chair and the child immediately darted for the chair and sat. The staff then rolled him out of the chaos and into a quiet space where he calmed down and went back to class without incident.

The story above is a prime example of how we can regulate the environment to either hinder or help a child. The staff in this scenario could have tried to physically intervene to stop this child, but considering he was over six feet tall and very athletically inclined, it would have taken several staff to stop him. Most likely he would have become more stressed and elevated if a physical intervention were to happen. In this case, a chair did the trick.

Color, light, and sound
Color

Colors are very important in the world of a child with autism because they can influence the child's state of emotional arousal and memory (Dzulkifli and Mustafar 2013). There are colors known to excite, such as red; conversely, there are colors that calm, such as the muted blues, greens, and grays (Elliot *et al.* 2007; Stone and English 1998). Red, bright yellows and highly reflective colors are excitatory and have their place in our world, but these are not the best colors to use for a child who is anxious or hyper-aroused at baseline. Temple Grandin helped design the homes for children with autism at The Center. She strongly suggested muted southwestern colors be used in these homes. Following her recommendation, we chose blue, green and pallets of pale oranges and yellows, which clearly have a calming affect for everyone.

Colors can also be used for wayfinding (i.e. helping the child find their way). You can actively reduce stress through wayfinding and at the same time increase independence during transitions. Designating certain colors to help a child find their way in a place can be very useful. For example, telling the child to follow the green square tiles on the floor to get to the lunch room or to go into the room with the yellow door for reading is a good use of color cueing.

Light

Light is also important for the child with autism. Natural light is a biological cue and important for maintaining circadian rhythms. Circadian rhythms are the 24-hour daily cycles in which we typically wake up, eat, work, eat, work, eat, relax, sleep, and wake up again. Although there are daily variations on our activities, as humans we follow a certain daily rhythm. Artificial light, such as light generated by some fluorescents, may interfere with circadian rhythms because it can suppress melatonin production. Melatonin is a natural hormone that helps regulate sleep and wake cycles. Fluorescent lights can also flicker and produce a low hum noise, which can be distracting, put strain on the eyes, and cause headaches (Rea 2000). I would recommend warm white bulbs in the environment instead of fluorescents in order to prevent melatonin suppression and to reduce other side effects.[1] These bulbs can be bought online—Cree 9.5 watt (60 watt), soft warm white (2700K) LED bulb.

I also highly recommend natural light whenever possible. If there is a glare, glare-reducing window shades can be used. Natural light can relax children and reduce hyperactivity (Brand, Dunn and Greb 2002). Natural light can also support improved academic performance (Fielding 2009; Mott *et al.* 2012). Many studies have demonstrated that sunlight and nature views can improve your overall health and mood, reduce stress, and actually reduce sick days—this applies to both children and adults.

Sound

Sound sensitivity has been well documented to be a problem in many children with autism. Children with sound sensitivities will often cue you by putting their fingers in their ears or perhaps even screeching or becoming aggressive when certain sounds are experienced. Typically these sensitivities are to select sounds and not all. I have heard from many parents that the first sign that they had that there was something amiss with their child was related to sound. In particular it was the sound of the vacuum that often resulted in their child having a meltdown. Sometimes installing sound soak on walls or adding a textured painting or carpet hung on a wall will help dampen sound. Area rugs on the floors can also really help to reduce sound coming from the external environments. These are good and relatively inexpensive ways to reduce acoustic noise.

---

1   http://beuth.de/de/technische-regel/din-spec-67600/170956045

Chemicals

Chemicals are used in many spaces for many reasons. One frequent use of chemicals is for cleaning the environment. Using chemicals, especially toxic cleaning products, in the home and school environments particularly for children with vulnerable neurological systems is not a good idea. Since you are working toward restoring health through this framework, adding toxins to the environment is simply counterproductive. I would recommend beginning to eliminate cleaners that contain harmful toxins and substituting them with natural cleaning products. This makes sense for anyone. None of us want to live in an environment that will poison us.

There is a section at the end of the book that lists products and recipes to make non-toxic cleaning solutions that are safe to use. I suggest beginning with the following few core ingredients that you can buy online or from your supermarket: baking soda, white distilled vinegar, lemon juice, washing soda, borax, and tea tree oil. You can save quite a lot of money using effective and easy to make homemade cleaning solutions. Compared to off-the-shelf cleaners in the grocery store, they are cheap and you avoid adding harmful products to the home environment. I always ask school personnel which cleaners they use, and encourage them to use non-toxic products as there are many children affected by strong chemicals and smells including those with asthma and other respiratory conditions.

If you are using chemicals bought off the shelf, read the labels before you purchase and store these in a child-proof, locked cabinet. If you are making your own cleaners, you can use the recipes at the end of the book or search for others online or in your local book store. Remember to always store chemicals, even if non-toxic, in a locked cabinet.

Transitioning from place to place

Transitioning from place to place can often be difficult for a child with autism for the many of the reasons discussed in earlier chapters. Children with autism can be overwhelmed by change especially if they are unsure about what is coming next.

When you are on the go, travelling, or visiting people in less than familiar spaces, it is sometimes helpful to bring a small, familiar object for the child. This could be a bean bag chair or sitting pillow. Having this object means that there will be an element of consistency for the child, even in foreign situations. Regardless of the room configuration the child will have their own space or place where they can relax and soak in the new environment.

I worked with one child who used to carry around a small blanket, and he actually put the blanket over his head in new spaces until he was ready to slowly take it off and experience the new space. It's really difficult and fatiguing for most children with autism to travel to new places. It requires a lot of focus, energy, and attention. Sometime it's helpful to use a pre-recorded video tour of a new space, such as a video tour of a hotel, shopping center or other public space that the child can view (as many times as needed) before traveling to the new place. The ability to know what the space looks like often helps decrease the associated stress and anxiety and increase understanding of what is expected.

The point is that children with autism are regulated or dysregulated by the external, physical environment. They seem to take in everything all at once. If the environment is highly disorganized and unpredictable, they will struggle and become stressed. Through years of my own observations coupled with the work of others observing and measuring physiological responses in children with autism, it's well established that transitioning from one activity/environment to the next can be very disorganizing and stressful for the child with autism. It is during these times that the stress "fight or flight" response can be activated.

For example, there are times when a child will drop to the ground during a transition from one place to another, and skilled behavioral staff observing the child may suggest that they are perhaps dropping to the ground to avoid the next activity. However, when viewing the child from the inside out using physiological monitoring, they may demonstrate signs of stress with increased heart rate and elevated EDA. When allowed to rest and to practice some self-calming techniques such as a deep breathing relaxation technique, as described in the chapter on emotional self-regulation, the child will calm down. The typical response is for the child to rest and then be able to proceed to the next activity.

Given the documented high rates of problems for children during transitions, I suggest instituting transitional benches for sitting that are either built in or placed outside of classrooms, in the entrance to homes, and in other high transitional areas. These are just resting benches. The use of these benches has been highly successful, and the children naturally and readily gravitate to them during transitional times. Once the child is sitting, the parent, clinician, or teacher can use a temporal, visual schedule to reaffirm the upcoming activity(s). This procedure helps to calm the child. Over time, they will learn to transition more easily.

Building a new environment

Building new includes being able to engage in construction to build from scratch. If the construction is commercial, such as a school, there are typically regulations and laws that include people with disabilities. Many of these adaptations or requirements are specifically designed for physical disabilities and some sensory disabilities. However, these may not be accommodating for some children with autism. There may be additional structural and material considerations that can be brought to bear to enhance social interaction, reduce stress, and promote health and well-being. These considerations include spatial design, color, sound, and light, and the use of green and organic building products and surfaces. I recommend reading the report funded by the Jeffrey Cook Trust for more detail on new models for living for young adults with autism. This report, A New Model for Shared Housing, was a joint project by The Center for Discovery staff and the Michael Singer Studio (2014) in response to the need for adult housing opportunities for autism and sustainable practices.

In addition to the built environment, the natural environment plays an important role in how children with autism function. The natural environment includes everything outdoors that is not a physical, man-made structure.

The natural outdoor environment

The beauty of the outdoors is that it doesn't have to be fancy nor does it have to be elaborate. It's amazing how children are able to create their own learning through play using rocks, trees, sand, sticks, and other natural items found in the outdoors.

The benefits of nature, trees, grasses, and green outdoor environments are well documented in the literature and known to support both the physical and mental health of everyone. The mental health benefits for children with autism are discussed in more detail in Chapter 6 on emotional regulation. In a report released by the City Parks Forum, a program of the American Planning Association (Frumkin and Eysenbach 2007), four key points describe the benefits of being in nature as follows:

1. Parks with trees and green spaces provide people with contact with nature, known to confer certain health benefits and enhance well-being.

2. Physical activity opportunities in parks help to increase fitness and reduce obesity.

3. Park resources can mitigate the effects of climate, air, and water pollution on public health.

4. Cities need to provide all types of parks, to provide their various citizen groups with a range of health benefits.

In children with attention deficit and in teens with behavioral disorders research findings suggest that contact with nature results in significant improvement in functioning and a reduction in behaviors (Frumkin 2001). It stands to reason that the same holds true for children with autism.

I am a strong advocate for the use of nature in teaching children with autism. There is mounting evidence demonstrating that outdoor learning is intrinsically motivating and boosts physical and mental activity (Broda 2011; Davies 1996; Kaiser Family Foundation 2010). Sometimes children who have autism who may not have elaborate play skills will just sit or roll on the grass enjoying the outdoor space in a casual way. Even this type of play can reduce stress and anxiety in children. If you live in a city, just taking a walk in a park can relieve daily stress.

Place-based learning

Place-based learning is often promoted in the literature as a great way to teach children because it takes advantage of the motivating natural landscape. This educational method uses natural objects such as rocks, water, trees, and leaves, and insects such as ants that children are most familiar with in order to teach basic skills and concepts. It's a natural and vicarious way to learn, and typically one that doesn't evoke a stress response because children are most familiar with and comfortable in their natural environment. I am a very strong proponent of place-based learning for children with autism. During place-based outdoor learning, social skill development is naturally easier as children are motivated and happier to be in these environments, and will more readily participate in social exchanges.

THE TEMPORAL ENVIRONMENT— THE TIMING AND ORDER OF THINGS

The temporal environment is the part of the environment that is constantly changing, and is based on time. Within the temporal environment, the timing and order of everything that happens is important for helping a child with autism feel safe, relaxed, and ready to learn. Because children with autism are often internally disorganized or dysregulated, activity-based or time-based picture/word schedules can really help reduce anxiety and promote calmness. Every child I have ever known with autism has benefited from an organized schedule whether it's a simple activity schedule or a portable web-based schedule. It takes off the pressure of not knowing what's coming next. If you think about it, we all use a schedule of sorts—a daily calendar is a time-based schedule, and as life becomes busier for all of us, schedules become even more important.

In this section, I will discuss the importance of routines, schedules, and structured activity with suggestions of best practice for all of these.

A structured and organized environment is one that establishes clear routines, rules, and timeframes for the child who has autism to successfully navigate through their day, from day to day, with the goal of preventing or reducing anxiety and stress (Hannah 2001). A good way to start is to begin thinking about the day in terms of chunks of time or activities—a school morning is a chunk that is probably made up of getting up, getting dressed and washed, eating breakfast, packing a book bag, and leaving the house for school. The actual transition to school, whether by walking, car, or bus is another chunk. The after school chunk may include a music lesson or a sport, or it may be homework or a leisure activity like watching TV or listening to music. Then there is the dinner chunk, followed by another activity again before preparing for bed.

Each of these activity chunks should be represented for the child in tangible, visual forms because they will respond better to this type of information than to simply being told what is going to happen. You can use either pictures or words including specific timeframes. Depending on how many activities they have, each of these chunks can be expressed in one schedule or multiple schedules.

Children who have autism process visual information more easily than verbal information (Ring *et al.* 1999). Visual information such as a written or picture-based schedule is permanent and concrete and can be easily referred to as many times as needed. Auditory information, once given, is gone unless it is recorded and can be replayed. When I teach people about the temporal dimension, I often use the analogy of being lost in a new country, sleep deprived and needing to find directions. I tell the audience to envision themselves in this scenario: to imagine and feel the stress that can occur under these circumstances. I ask them to then visualize themselves approaching a stranger in this foreign country to ask for directions. Hopefully that stranger speaks their language. If the directions that are given to them are verbal and are more than two steps, they will most likely forget them if they don't write them down.

Stressed brains cannot remember. Even if they ask to have the directions repeated two to three times, when they walk away, within several minutes, they will most likely forget what was said.

In my experience, the audience can become stressed just visualizing themselves in the scenario, which helps them to imagine what a child with autism might experience in a situation with an overload of information. This scenario is not unlike what happens to children with autism, except for them life can be like living in a foreign country every day—even if they experience the same scenario every day. Sometimes a child can become overwhelmed by the circumstances of the day and how they are feeling.

There are many external and internal factors that can affect children from day to day, and it's important to add supports and even decrease expectations if the child is having a difficult day. For example, external factors might include the number of people in the environment, the time of day, or the location of the event. Internal factors could include whether the child slept that night, if they are constipated or have loose stools, or had a seizure, for example. Trying to coax the child into behaving better using candy or other rewards, although tempting for many parents and teachers, is not the best solution.

On some days in our school program, we have seen children who are able to complete a routine request without much prompting. On other days, when their stress level is high per their EDA, they have great difficulty understanding what is expected of them even during a typical routine. These are the days that additional supports for the child are very important. Additional supports could be giving them extra time and/or additional visual cues. You may need to be much more explicit in your directions and allow for greater processing time. On these kinds of days, problems may also be exacerbated if you provide too much information all at once. These are also the times when you should look for other potential problems that can be upsetting to the child. Problems might include medical or biological concerns that come from lack of sleep or having a stomachache or not feeling well in general.

Reading body language as a clue

Trina, a mom of a 22-year-old with a complex form of autism, would often share with me that she could tell immediately by looking in her son's eyes if the day was going to be good or bad. If his pupils were dilated and he was wide eyed, she knew immediately not to push him. It just wouldn't be worth the fight that would inevitably ensue. She could tell that something was not right, and the problem was typically medical, a pre-seizure response, or it could be stemming from his routine being out of the norm. She also knew that less was more in terms of what she said to him. He just couldn't listen too much on these days. He needed short directives, without repeating them, and ample time to process what she said. She knew that he heard her when he switched the conversation and started talking about Europe—his favorite map place. Her advice for other parents was patience and more patience. Parents should learn to read body language and facial expressions and be ready to adjust their expectations on certain days.

Structured approaches

An overall structured approach uses visual (written materials or pictures) and physical supports and strategies to communicate directions, which include daily schedules, expected interactions, physical boundaries, and spatial relationships. Organized learning spaces provide concrete visual information and address challenging behaviors in a proactive, anticipatory manner by creating appropriate and meaningful environments that should reduce the stress, anxiety, and frustration often experienced by children with autism (Stokes 2003). Environmental cues, such as physical and/or color-coded room boundaries, designate specific functions of an area. Children feel secure when they understand their boundaries and expectations. Initially, children's individual spaces may be color coded or distinctly labeled, or their names may be used as a cue about the location of their space relative to another child's and to the larger environment. Sometimes it is helpful to use colored duct tape to distinguish the child's space relative to another's space. By clearly indicating spaces and spatial relationships, a child can focus on relevant information and what they are expected to do or learn.

Time-sequenced schedules, when clearly communicated, can help children perform tasks and activities without direct prompting and guidance by parents or teachers (McClannahan and Krantz 1997). Precise and detailed time-based schedules are critical to a structured and systematic teaching approach. They are designed with a child's skill level, physical ability, preferences, age, attention span, and endurance in mind. For example, a schedule may be designed using object cues presented in a top to bottom format with five objects visible at once. Another schedule may use picture icons in a left to right format with two picture icons visible at once. The visual presentation of the schedule allows the child to see what is happening in the present moment and to anticipate what will come next. This will help reduce stress and anxiety. For beginners, I highly recommend communicating visually what is happening in the moment, and only what is to happen next. This is sometimes referred to as "first/ then" schedule. During transitions, tools such as verbal countdowns (5 – 4 – 3 – 2 – 1, go), timers, and count down strips (numbers displayed in descending order) can be used to avoid behavioral overreactions that can occur with change or from a lack of understanding of the concept of time.

Activities

In order to keep children engaged and to encourage them to initiate participation in an activity, activities should be based as much as possible on preferences and experiences. Activities should be presented in a way that incorporates structure and organization as required for each child. A strong focus on the process of learning rather than simply completing the task allows for more spontaneous interactions and lifelong learning skills.

For instance, let's look at the lesson of learning to grow a tomato from a seed, which can be used to teach organizational skills. If the task is to learn to grow a tomato, the end result might be harvesting and eating the tomato, which is great. However, along the journey of growing the tomato there are many ways to enhance the child's learning. Since planting a tomato requires a series of actions, teach the use of making pictures or word cards to sequence the actions of the task of planting. This might include making a picture of a pot, then a picture of soil being added to the pot, then a picture of a seed, and lastly a picture of a water jug. These pictures together highlight the major actions in this simple activity. Helping the child to make the pictures is a lifelong skill that teaches the child how to think through and organize their thoughts. I work with a child who has poor fine motor skills and doesn't like to draw. Instead of drawing, he takes pictures of the steps, prints the pictures, and then puts them in his notebook in the correct sequence.

The next step in the process of planting a tomato is the creation of a calendar to be used to remind the child of when to water the plant. The exercise can help a child understand the concept of a calendar and how to make one, which is a lifelong skill that applies to almost everything we do. I recommend stocking up on calendars and keeping them in all major areas where activities happen. If the child is skilled in using electronic calendars, one computer tablet can hold all the calendars. Next in the planting scenario is the creation of a journal to document the progress of the seed as it transforms into a plant and ultimately bears fruit. Sequencing and journal documenting are lifelong skills that support the child with autism in everyday functioning. Journaling can be used for many activities; the act of journaling about a potentially stressful event before it occurs can reduce the level of stress a child might experience from that event (Beilock 2015).

These steps for the process of planting have value and can be applied to many other tasks the child will complete during their day and also during their lifetime. Like creating a time-based activity schedule, all lesson-based activities can be broken down into a sequence of tasks using explicit visual cues that can indicate what action is expected and how the task is to be organized. These kinds of activities together help to reduce stress on the child as they learn to navigate expectations and interactions.

Multitasking

Multitasking or being able to do multiple activities simultaneously is really a misnomer. As much as we think that we can multitask, according to Beilock (2015) our brains can't really multitask. Only 1 percent of the total population can actually perform simultaneous processing such that their brains can fully attend to two separate inputs at once. For the remaining 99 percent of us, we need to stop one input before attending to another. In other words, in order to be fully focused on one activity, we need to completely stop any other activities that might distract us.

Many studies born out of the texting craze have now demonstrated that it's just not possible for the brain to type or read and still attend to the environment. It's why texting and driving has now been outlawed in so many countries. For children with autism, multitasking is really not possible. They can't discriminate what to pay attention to, and they are trying to pay attention to everything. It's as though their brains are attempting to multitask all the time. In response, their stress levels elevate when there is too much stimulation. To help children with autism to be successful, it is best to present them with one task at a time, and be clear and concise with expectations using temporal cueing, which is described in the next section.

THE SOCIAL ENVIRONMENT

Part of the hallmark of having autism is having difficulty in social situations, including having poor social understanding and perception, and poor communication skills both verbal and nonverbal. One of the major problems for children with autism as a result of poor social skills is that they may not have friends or they may have difficulty maintaining friendships.

The Easter Seals Study (Easter Seals 2008) revealed that 79 percent of children with autism are living at home beyond 18, and only 17 percent of those had a friend in the community. It's really important to begin to teach children to interact with others, especially how to make and keep friends. According to Frankel, there are many positive benefits in social skills training that lead to improved social interaction and peer relationships (Frankel *et al.* 2010). I recommend using a program such as Reciprocal Imitation Training (RIT), designed by Brooke Ingersoll, Ph.D. (Berger and Ingersoll 2013) from the University of Michigan researched in a study with participants at The Center for Discovery (Ingersoll *et al.* 2013). I will describe the critical components of this program in this section, but in teaching social skills or in finding an appropriate social program, based on experience, I look for a variety of developmentally appropriate programs that have the following qualities:

* gradually and systematically teaches new social experiences—building a library of experiences that are repeated often and expanded upon

* has rules of social events clearly spelled out—such as how to act in a movie theater, at a birthday party, at the dinner table, etc… and, encourages reviews of these rules often

* helps guide the child through social events with cues about expectations and next steps, and slowly decreases supports when they are comfortable

* uses plays, dramas, music, and other social grouping activities that are scripted to help the child understand all the different ways to interact

* provides direct instruction on using and understanding facial expressions and gestures, starting and stopping conversations, imitating, and interrupting conversations

* uses stories, movie clips, or video-modeling to teach emotional content.

Reciprocal imitation training (RIT)

RIT can be used to get the child started in social skill development. It is often difficult to teach social skills to children who have more complex forms of autism because they have difficulty grasping and understanding the concept of interaction. Recognizing and understanding which skills to employ in different situations is complex. Education programs are usually focused on teaching imitation, wherein the child is asked to look at others, appropriately greet others, and learn to take turns.

Imitation is often considered difficult to teach because it is challenging to get the child's attention and even harder to sustain it. However, imitation is essential because it's actually how children begin to learn to interact with others and to jointly attend to an activity. The goal of looking at another will only happen in earnest if the child is interested in the other person. Looking at another person for an M&M just isn't the same.

Research suggests that children with autism have particular difficulty imitating in unstructured social settings. Interventions that can teach spontaneous imitation skills during natural interactions may be effective for promoting flexible, social imitation and other social-communication skills (Ingersoll *et al.* 2013). Learning to imitate is an essential long-term life skill and is one that will lead to establishing friendships.

RIT is a natural intervention that occurs during play and in daily routines. What's important about the program is that it can be taught with minimal instruction by a parent, teacher, or other support personnel. The goal is to teach imitation as means of social interaction with the child imitating the actions of the adult or peer. The actual accuracy of the performance of the action is less important. What matters is that the child attempts to imitate, which confirms that they are noticing what the other person is doing, and desire to do the same. Essentially it demonstrates that the child wants to interact with another person. This is foundational for all social development.

The RIT technique uses several strategies to teach imitation and it has been proven to be effective with young children and adolescents who have autism. It can be taught in a variety of settings and used during daily routines. It's been our experience that even children with significant maladaptive behaviors and children who are very distractible can learn to imitate others. According to Carlsen, an RIT instructor at The Center for Discovery, as the child progresses in skills, they appear calmer and often are generally more focused. This program can be used with any child who is not consistent in imitative skills. And, the good news is that it's never too late to begin to teach social skills. Actually, it's imperative that children learn how to interact successfully with others in ways that are positive and that decrease stress and anxiety—whether they are 3 or 33. There is a simple guidebook of how to teach imitation using this method that can be found online or by searching online for Reciprocal Imitation Training, pdf.[2]

Friendships

You don't need a lot of friends to be psychologically and emotionally happy. It seems that most children with autism want to have friends and friendships, but may experience difficultly developing and maintaining those friendships. Some of the reasons may be restricted interest, lack of advanced social and

---

2   https://ieccwa.org/uploads/IECC2014/HANDOUTS/KEY_2720064/
     RITManual.pdf

language skills, and/or delayed cognitive skills. It can be a matter of geography that makes maintaining friendships difficult. For instance, if you live in a very rural setting where there are fewer children around and/or people live in homes that are farther apart it may be more difficult to find and meet with friends.

In order to foster a friendship, the first step is to pair children who have similar interests. This can happen during school, during a community activity, or in the home setting. The pairing may be to complete school assignments or to participate in cooperative community activities. Activities that are motivating, which require interactions like building or producing something, are the best types of activities to begin to foster friendships. An example might be building a sandcastle, a tree fort (even a living room fort), an ice sculpture, a Lego structure—anything that requires cooperation and joint attention, just use your imagination. Or, it may simply be putting two children together who like to bounce balls where you are working on taking turns with the ball. Friendships are fostered and will grow by spending more time together, so you need to work at keeping time set aside for developing a friendship. It's really important for overall health and well-being, especially mental health. It's well documented that having friends reduces stress and even increases life expectancy.

One of the children I work with articulated that his first real friend at age 16 was a boy who used to tie his shoes for him. He was very happy to have a friend even though the interaction was limited to shoe tying. Amazingly it was so positive for his emotional state that it encouraged him to try to have more friends. Sometimes it's the positive first experiences in friendships that invite us and encourage us to continue to learn to interact. Today that same young man has several good friends. He can and will tell you all the things that he does with his friends such as just hang out, play games, go out to eat, watch football, and have parties. He understands the social and emotional value of having a friend.

We can guide the interactions of the child with autism by setting up the opportunities for interaction. It's an additive concept—you start simple and add complexity to the interactions as you progress. I recommend using RIT to introduce imitation that can be used in interaction; then add a coaching component to help the child learn how to expand the interaction in real time.

An example is that you might provide the child with directions for how to approach a peer. You could give them a detailed, written script that you can practice together before the actual interaction. To help the child better understand the script, you can create flash cards with a picture to illustrate each step of the interaction. Here is a possible scripted interaction:

1. Walk up to the child you want to be friends with.

2. Wait to get their attention or say "Hi" to get their attention.

3. Smile and make eye contact.

4. Ask, "Can I play?" or "Would you like to play together on X day?"

Practice this simple interaction at home or with small groups of familiar people several times until the child is ready to reach out to someone they are less familiar with—the child they want to become friends with. Observe the interaction; as appropriate, comment on how the child did using real examples and positive, provisional language. For example:

> "Your eye contact was good, and the length of time you maintained eye contact was also good. Next time, you may want to say Hi to get (child's name) attention, rather than standing there without saying anything. Give the child a strategy like: try counting to 5, and if (child's name) doesn't stop and look at you, you can interrupt by saying Hi. Now, let's practice this."

The first time may not always be successful, so it's important to continue to learn from each experience and keep offering positive feedback. Over time, the child will become more and more comfortable with those first and most difficult interactions. Practice and make it fun—you should never be at a loss of variations on social interactions to practice. Remember, one good friend is enough to make all the difference in someone's life.

Social stories

Social stories are visual tools that can be used to teach concepts, skills, or desired behaviors for social situations. Creating simple social stories or social cartoons is a great way to encourage social connectedness and engagement, and to teach improved understanding of upcoming events and expectations. There is a tremendous amount of information already available about social stories. I recommend going right to the source—Carol Gray's website—for great examples.[3]

Social stories are effective because the information presented is highly relevant, orderly, focused, structured, and presented in a visual format. The latter may be the most important because children with autism seem to respond very positively to visual learning techniques. All of these are critical components for a child with autism to learn. The stories can be simple with many pictures and few words, or more complex and lengthy, which makes them accessible for all levels of development and functioning. For older children, social articles can be written at an age-appropriate level and format.

Creating social stories together with your child is a great activity, as it reinforces sequencing of events and it creates structure to social events and interactions. Because the social milieu is always changing, there are endless iterations of possible stories that you can create. You can think about creating social

---

3   www.thegraycenter.org/social-stories/what-are-social-stories

stories together as a nightly or weekend activity. In so doing, you are helping your child develop a long-term, lifelong skill, while also spending quality, healthy time with them.

StoryScape

There are many effective ways to teach social skills including ones that take advantage of technology. One example is StoryScape, which is an online, free program.

Online programs can be very effective as an educational learning method for children with autism. StoryScape is a promising open source, free online program that has been trialed at The Center for Discovery. StoryScape was created by Eckhardt, Ferguson and Picard (2013) from the MIT Media Lab affective computing group. It's a highly interactive and animated platform designed to promote English-Language-Arts (ELA) skill acquisition, and it is also turning out to be a powerful social emotional platform that can be used to teach empathy and emotional regulation. StoryScape was developed to motivate children to interact with others by creating group-based stories using a fun, easy digital platform. Teachers who have used the platform are reporting significant increases in student participation, attention, and on-task behavior. The results demonstrate that the children who have used this program are more social with increased interactions with others. I highly recommend this program for teachers to use with children in the classroom and also for families to use as an interactive tool with their child at home. Best of all, it's free and can be found by searching online for "StoryScape."

SUMMARY

The environment—including the physical, temporal, and social dimensions where the child lives, learns, and plays—is very important to their overall health and well-being. Take time to reflect on the areas presented in this chapter, and identify one thing that you could regulate that may make your child's life easier today. I encourage you to make that adjustment or change and keep a journal of what works and what doesn't. Not everything will work; sometimes, it just takes time and patience. A word of caution—don't take on too much at once; start small and build up gradually so that you can set yourself and the child up for success.

Self-assessment

It's time to re-evaluate your knowledge in understanding how the environment can be regulated to either help or hinder a child with autism and to note one thing that you might want to try during the next week or so.

ENVIRONMENT

1   4   7

Little knowledge   *Very knowledgeable*

One thing I would like to try:

_____

Chapter 5

EATING
AND NUTRITION
REGULATION

Theresa Hamlin
with Jennifer Frank, RD

This chapter is about food, eating, and nutrition. The quality and quantity of what children eat is really important to their health, vitality, and ability to learn and manage stress. Food is also important to you as a parent who is facing extraordinary challenges raising a child with autism.

You may find comfort in knowing that no one has it all together when it comes to food. Some of us are waiting for the 3-D printer to design and cook our food at will, while others would just like food to be in a pill form. However, there are basics that we all should know when it comes to providing healthy diets for our children and ourselves. This chapter will introduce you to these basics and will include research that illustrates why quality food is important for children with autism.

The first question to explore is how the food we eat can affect our stress levels and health. The intestine or gut is directly connected to the brain by a pipeline that allows communication between the two. A lot of this is accomplished through very important components of both the gut and brain called neurotransmitters. What we eat and how we digest our food essentially affects how we think. The stomach or gut is now being referred to as the body's second brain, thanks to the work of Michael Gershon (1998), prominent neuroscientist at Columbia University Medical Center and author of the book *The Second Brain*. According to Gershon, upon eating, the gut sends messages directly to the brain via the vagus nerve pathway and through the bloodstream. Via the brain, the gut can control how much you sleep, how much energy you have, your emotional state, and your sense of well-being (Mayer and Tillisch 2011). The gut is also responsible for breaking down all of the foods that you eat, absorbing good nutrients, and eliminating wastes that are not useful to the body and can sometimes be harmful. Thus bowel movements are important to pay attention to as they give us clues into the body's digestive health.

Studies have shown that there are some foods that increase stress levels and other that may act as elixirs when a body is under stress. There are also certain foods that enhance the availability of serotonin in the brain. Serotonin is known to have a calming effect and helps with sleep.

According to Dr. Kara Gross Margolis, pediatric gastroenterologist and neuroscientist at the Columbia University Medical Center and also part of The Center for Discovery research team, there is a highly significant association between gastrointestinal (GI) problems, serotonin and difficult behaviors like aggression and self-injury. Margolis has also noted that about 95 percent of the body's serotonin is found in the bowels, and is studying the effect of serotonin on the gut in children with autism. Interestingly, serotonin plays critical roles in how fast or slow the gut moves, and issues with gut motility may be contributing to issues like chronic constipation and diarrhea.

In 2013, a groundbreaking study using lab mice demonstrated that feeding mice bacteria known as Bacteriodesfragilits, a microbe known to bolster the immune system, actually reduced the aberrant behaviors seen in autistic mice (Hsiao *et al.* 2013). Researchers are also finding that gut microbes may also impact a person's cognition, emotion, and mental health (Gilbert *et al.* 2013). There are many other studies currently underway examining the effects of different probiotics in restoring the gut flora including ones that lower the hormone cortisol.

According to McEwen and Lasley (2002), laboratory animals that are fed a high-fat and processed food diet have higher cortisol levels. The negative effects of cortisol were discussed in Chapter 2; those high levels take significantly longer to return to baseline when the animals are subjected to stress. What seems clear from this study and others like it is that there are certain foods that support health and vitality and there are other foods that can negatively affect health and vitality. Some foods can lead to weight gain, lack of sleep, and ultimately a vicious cycle of stress, while foods containing Omega 3 fatty acids, folate, B vitamins, and/or low glycemic foods can improve mood and decrease anxiety (Perica and Delas 2011; Ross 2009).

FOOD—A NATIONAL HEALTH PRIORITY IN AUTISM

In 2010, research on GI functioning and eating problems for children with autism became a priority for the National Institute of Health Interagency Autism Coordinating Committee (2014). Data reported from the Autism Treatment network showed that 50 percent of individuals participating in 14 identified academic health centers had GI problems. Those with GI problems were more likely to have sleep problems, behavioral problems, and lower health-related quality of life.

Buie and colleagues (Buie *et al.* 2010) and Coury (2010) have indicated that the assessment and treatment of GI problems can improve functioning and quality of life. There is evidence that an atypical pattern of eating in children with autism places them at risk for long-term nutritional and medical complications not captured by broad measures including vitamin and mineral deficiencies.

The Department of Pediatrics at Emory University School of Medicine and research staff at the Marcus Center conducted a meta-analysis in 2013. The study revealed that children with autism had lower intake of calcium and protein and a higher number of nutrient deficits overall. Food selectivity, and other atypical patterns of eating for children with autism, often included excessive consumption of processed and calorie-dense foods. The results of this type of selective eating behavior can lead to obesity and increased body and brain stress (Monthly International Autism Magazine 2013).

Mazurek and colleagues (Mazurek *et al.* 2013) demonstrated that GI problems were linked with high anxiety and regression in behavior. Once the GI problems were treated, the anxiety and regression ceased. As noted in the study, psychotropic drugs, which are a common treatment for anxiety and maladaptive behaviors, could actually make the GI conditions worse in some children.

Scientists at Columbia University's Mailman School for Public Heath recently conducted a large longitudinal study, confirming that children with ASDs were two and half times more likely to experience persistent GI symptoms as infants and toddlers than their peers (Bresnahan *et al.* 2015).

Another recent meta-analysis of 15 studies revealed that children with ASD experience significantly more GI symptoms than their peers and have higher rates of diarrhea, constipation, and abdominal pain (McElhanon *et al.* 2014). Tim Buie (2015), M.D. and gastroenterologist and researcher from Harvard University Medical School, noted that GI problems are not just part of autism and that they occur at high rates in children with autism and must be treated medically. Food is an important factor in that treatment.

GASTROINTESTINAL AND FOOD PROBLEMS
FIRST DESCRIBED BY KANNER

In his descriptions of children with autism, Dr. Leo Kanner (1943) noted that nearly all of the children had undiagnosed gastrointestinal and eating problems. Many children had severe eating problems from the very beginning of life. Here are some of the children's parents' statements:

> Eating has always been a problem for him. He has never shown a normal appetite. (p.217)

> He vomited a great deal during the first year. Had to be tube fed until 1 year of age. (p.244)

> The main thing that worries me is the difficulty in feeding. That is the essential thing, and secondly his slowness in development. (p.237)

> For the first two months the feeding formula caused considerable concern. (p.233)

> He vomited all food from birth through the third month. (p.31)

At the time Dr. Kanner was writing about these problems, they were thought to be psychogenic and were attributed to a psychiatric issue rather than a biological or physiological problem. Thankfully, the science around these problems, especially GI problems, has progressed significantly. We now understand that there are clear physical and/or medical problems in children with autism associated with food, eating, and digestion.

Despite the abundance of new scientific information from recent studies, we still hear from parents that their child's GI problems are viewed either as just another part of having autism or as a behavioral component of autism and thus not treated.

GI PROBLEMS ARE UNIVERSAL

Dr. Buie and I were both invited to Saudi Arabia in 2014 for a conference on autism in Onaizah. During our opening session, it was evident that there was great concern from professionals about the eating behavior of children with autism, as well as possible GI problems resulting from this behavior. Many children reportedly had highly self-restricted diets that consisted primarily of processed foods. There was also a concern from many of the teachers about the children's behaviors and the use of candy as a motivator or reward to control behavior. The teachers seemed better informed and aware that the candy in the long run was not the best option to help the children; however, like many professionals, they were unclear about other options and were seeking advice. After my time in Saudi Arabia, I traveled to Al Ain and Dubai to hear the very same concerns about poor diets that echoed what we hear in the United States. It was clear to me that the problems around food were universal and of great concern to parents and professionals. I have come to believe that food and eating deserves national and international attention and further research.

The critical message for parents and professionals is that, because of the well-documented relationships between food, stress, and GI problems, food should be considered to be a form of health care. What we eat has the power to heal us and also the power to make us sick. In other words, what a child puts in their mouth should be helpful to their brain and body. Think about the fact that the three most critical activities that we must do every day to stay alive are to sleep, breathe, and eat. If the air we breathe, the amount that we sleep, and the food we eat are not helpful to our body for maintaining and building health, then nothing else really matters. It's the basis for survival, and the stronger and healthier we are, the better the outcome we will have as we navigate through all of life's challenges.

BOWEL MOVEMENTS: WHY THEY MATTER

Bowel movements are one of the first things to examine if GI issues are suspected. Considering the high rate of GI problems in children with autism, it is important to discuss bowel movements, which are the body's ability to eliminate waste. The size, color, and consistency of stool can reveal a great deal about a person's health, GI functioning, and digestion. The Bristol Stool Chart is a universal tool used to categorize bowel movements, with type 4 on the chart being the "best" and 3s and 5s being fairly common.

Ideally, children should move their bowels daily, perhaps even as often as three times per day. Every other day is also considered to be in the normal range. Diarrhea occurs when your intestine doesn't have time to absorb water from your stool because it passes so quickly through the digestive track. When it happens, diarrhea can be a sign of illness. Having chronic diarrhea, even once a week, is not normal and can be an indicator that something is wrong with the GI system. Should this situation arise, notify a doctor right away.

Conversely, constipation, which is hard and dry stool, usually occurs when there is decreased elimination. Chronic constipation can be painful and can lead to serious problems, like fecal impaction or the development of a mega-colon. Both chronic constipation and diarrhea should be brought to the attention of a physician. They are not part of an autism diagnosis but are seen at high rates in children with autism, who should be medically evaluated if they experience one or the other or both.

The health of your stomach, intestines, and bowels are very important, as they have a direct influence on the brain's functioning and help to regulate stress and emotions. The health of your stomach is highly influenced by the food you eat and your ability to rid the body of waste.

FAST FOODS AND PROCESSED FOODS

It's well established that a balanced diet of quality whole foods can promote overall health and well-being. To the contrary, processed foods, especially those high in sugar and artificial ingredients, can contribute to obesity and lifelong health problems. Foods that are processed, as well as those that contain additives, can act as inflammatory agents in the body, which can lead to chronic health problems. Eating poor quality foods can exacerbate existing conditions such as stress, anxiety, GI and immune problems, behavioral difficulties, and sleep problems. These are the problems typically seen in children with autism that can be made worse by the foods they eat.

The dissection of a popular food for children

A recent study about the composition of chicken nuggets, a highly popular child's food, demonstrated that chicken was not a major component of the nugget. So what was in the chicken nugget? Nuggets that were examined from two popular fast food restaurants contained between 40–50 percent skeletal muscle and the rest was primarily fat with some blood and nerves. There was very little actual chicken meat in the nugget, which was simply not a very nutritious meal for a child (deShazo, Bigler and Baldwin-Skipworth 2013).

I bring this to your attention because as a society, and certainly as busy parents, we want to believe that what we buy in the grocery store and in restaurants is healthy for our children. We trust in others. However, foods that we think are healthy may not always be as they seem. For children who already have vulnerable systems and highly restrictive, self-imposed diets, the problem of eating unhealthy foods can exacerbate an already potentially dangerous situation.

Over the years, we have heard countless numbers of parents and teachers tell us that their child with autism just loves

M&Ms, French fries, macaroni and cheese, and chicken nuggets. We have no doubt that this is true. The problem is that this is *all* they like. They eat these foods at the exclusion of vegetables and other high nutrient types of foods. As a result, over time these children grow completely out of nutritional balance. This trend can unfortunately lead a child on a collision course toward chronic health problems.

Food as a reward

In the typical population of children, and also adults, a healthy balanced diet is very important for long-term health. It stands to reason that a healthy diet is even more important for children with autism. It appears, however, that not everyone treating children with autism views food with the same level of knowledge and priority. In April 2014, our local newspaper featured an article about a school district that had implemented a "state of the art" autism program. In the article, the teacher and Program Director were quoted as describing a new method of positive reinforcement. According to the Director, the new method "rewards the kids with a cookie only if they showed positive behavior, such as when they say, 'sit down, sit down,' and the child sits." Cookies were being used as a behavioral method to coax children to behave.

The method of using food rewards, multiple times per day, would never be encouraged for typically developing children, especially with obesity rates at epidemic proportions. So why is it allowable for the population of children who have autism? I remember my mother telling us as kids that we couldn't have a sweet food too close to dinner, or it would ruin our appetite. She always made sure that we ate breakfast, lunch, and dinner. My parents valued good food and nutrition, even though they knew nothing about organics. At the time, this just seemed like common sense. I passed this tradition on to my own children.

So, how is it that school staff and other professionals allow common sense to go out the window for children with autism?

What some educators may not understand is that a steady diet of foods made of sugar and other artificial ingredients significantly contributes to poor health and poor behavior. Ultimately, it contributes to the very same poor behavior that they were trying to eliminate in the first place. For children with autism, eating treats and sweets results in a downward spiral of health and functioning brought on by increased stress on the brain and body. Food as a contingency is problematic on many levels. Most importantly, it sets the child up with a poor relationship with food contributing to unhealthy eating habits resulting in further stress on the body. If a contingency for good behavior is needed, it is far better to use something that is not food related, such as increased play time, time using the computer, time in the gym, or running outdoors, which is by far a favorite for many children.

WHAT CAN YOU EAT?

What you put in your mouth to eat is often based on culture, personal preference, and what you know your body can tolerate. Nutritional science is continually evolving and changing, so what was recommended a decade ago as being healthy might not be the same as what is recommended today. There is, however, solid research about the foundations for promoting good health, disease-preventing foods, and ways to eat. So, let's discuss some of the "what to eat" recommendations.

The great news is that the best diet for your child is also what is best for you—a wholefoods, mostly plant-based diet, featuring as much pasture-raised, organic animal product and healthy fat as possible. What does that mean? Well, let's break it down.

Whole foods are the opposite of processed foods. They are foods in their natural state—no processing has been done to them and there is nothing added and nothing taken away. These are foods that have only a handful of ingredients that you should be able to recognize on the label—or even better—foods that don't have a label such as fresh fruits and vegetables. Plant based means you can find it growing on a farm or in the wild. It's usually a fruit, vegetable, or legume. When a food is plant based, it means that it is edible and comes from the ground or grows on a plant that is rooted in the ground.

In order to teach children about whole foods, it's sometimes worth a trip to the grocery store. You can find most of the whole foods in the vegetable, fruit, meat, and poultry aisles. These are typically aisles on the outer perimeter of the market because they require refrigeration and electricity that comes from the walls of the store. Shop the perimeter. This method is not always foolproof, however. Some fruits, vegetables, meats, and poultry in these aisles are laced with pesticides and other chemicals used to make these foods more appealing and heartier.

For fruits and vegetables, organic is usually best to buy as the conventional pesticides used to protect these products have been linked to a number of health woes including attention deficit hyperactivity disorder (Bouchard *et al.* 2010). However, if this is not possible for you, then try to buy what is in season and what is grown locally. Food that is grown locally is often fresher as it has not traveled across the country or around the world. Food loses vital nutrients each day that it sits in a warehouse or travels in a truck. If buying food in season or locally isn't possible, try to stick with fresh or frozen over canned. Canned foods often contain many preservatives that aren't compatible with our metabolism. The bottom line is that you want whole and real foods as much as possible. Luckily, many grocery stores are now increasing their stock as more as more people become aware of the health benefits of these foods.

Best and worst foods

The Environmental Working Group Shopper's Guide (2015) contains a list of fruits and vegetables that have the highest concentrations of chemicals, such as pesticides. Whenever possible, this is where I would advise buying organic. Remember, if organic isn't possible, stick with whole and real.

Buy organic—WORST FOODS (when not organic)	Lowest in pesticides— CLEANEST FOODS
Apples	Asparagus
Celery	Avocados
Cherries	Bananas
Grapes (imported)	Broccoli
Lettuce	Cabbage
Nectarines	Kiwi
Peaches	Mangos
Pears	Onions
Potatoes	Papaya
Spinach	Pineapples
Strawberries	Sweet corn, frozen
Sweet bell peppers	Sweet peas, frozen

Ten brain foods for children

Drew Ramsey, coauthor of *The Happiness Diet* (Graham and Ramsey 2011), suggests that there are ten essential foods that our children require for a healthy brain. The effects of eating these foods can last well into adulthood. His list consists of the following:

* eggs—contain nutrients including choline, Omega 3s, zinc, and lutein, which can help with attention

* greek yogurt—contain essential full fats, which is important for cell membrane health

* greens—nutrients include folate and vitamins, especially spinach and kale, which helps with new brain cell growth

* purple cauliflower—contains folate and B6 and has anti-inflammatory nutrients

* fish—contains vitamin D and Omega 3s, especially salmon, tuna, and sardines, which protect against cognitive decline

* animal meat—meat that is pasture raised without antibiotics or pesticides

* nuts and seeds—contain essential proteins, fatty acids, vitamins, and minerals, which help protect the nervous system

* oatmeal—contains essential proteins and fiber, which help with heart and brain health

* apples and plums—contain the antioxidants quercetin, which fights cognitive decline

* turmeric—a spice that contains curcumin, which is important for brain growth and contains essential anti-inflammatory properties; it's a natural compound that has been extensively researched and usually can be found in the spice aisle of your local grocery store.

There are many ways to begin to help your child become interested in healthy foods. One way is to get them to be part of the discovery of learning what is healthy and what is not so healthy. Your school health teacher may have strategies that can help. One strategy is to become a nutrition detective.

Getting your child involved in choosing healthy foods

"Nutrition Detectives" a really fantastic, free online program created by Katz *et al.* (2011) that is designed to teach all children how to make healthy food choices. It's a 90-minute program that comes with a PowerPoint and hands-on activities that you can complete with your child. It is easily adaptable for children with autism, as it uses lots of pictures and is sequential. The program offers five "clues" that help children think about the nutritional content of their food before they eat it. The clues are easy to understand:

1. Don't be fooled by the front of the package—look at the ingredients.

2. The first ingredient listed is the biggest!—the food has the most of this ingredient.

3. Avoid food with ingredients that don't belong—the things that aren't foods.

4. Avoid foods with a long ingredient list—more than 5 is usually not good.

5. Fiber is your friend! Beware of whole grain imposters.

The five concepts can be taught gradually. The child can take on the exciting role of being a detective in discovering what healthy foods look and taste like.

Katz *et al.* (2011) conducted a study to evaluate more than 1180 second through fourth graders enrolled in the Nutrition Detective program and found a significant increase in food label literacy compared to their aged-matched counterparts who were not exposed to the program. Along these lines, we have noticed that when a child with autism gets focused on healthy foods, they influence everyone around them to start to eat healthy as well! It is worth the effort to engage your child in understanding the difference between healthy and unhealthy eating. You can begin the program with a social story about healthy foods and then progress to reading labels and eventually to determining menus for creating healthy meals.[1]

---

1   The manual and program materials can be downloaded free of charge from: www.turnthetidefoundation.org/NutritionDetectives.aspx

TYPES OF DIETS AND OTHER PRODUCTS

There are literally hundreds, if not thousands, of different types of diets promoted by people from a wide spectrum of beliefs and backgrounds. However, when it comes to children, especially those with vulnerable systems, an informed, commonsense approach is best. This section will explore some of the basics when it comes to diets.

Plant-based diet

Plant based means that the majority of the diet should be made up of plant-based foods such as vegetables, fruits, and potentially some whole grains. If it makes it easier to imagine, think of the majority of the contents of your plate as being comprised primarily of fruits and vegetables. This is the diet that we recommend for children with autism to ensure that are getting a healthy nutrient-dense diet. We know, however, that this is not the diet that most children with autism are currently eating, but don't be discouraged if the thought of seeing your child eat a vegetable seems like a distant dream. Changing food and nutrition patterns takes months and sometimes years. This is a marathon, but one that your child will ultimately benefit from throughout their entire life. We work every day at helping children transition to a wholefoods diet—and it can still take months before those foods are readily accepted. The idea that a child will put a new food to their mouth, eat it, and enjoy it the first or second time around is not realistic for most; it may take time for them to even tolerate a food in the room or on the table. More about how to get a child to eat a balanced diet can be found later in this chapter.

I want to take a moment to mention a couple recent findings regarding grains and carbohydrates. Nutritional studies have been focusing on grains and gluten as potentially problematic for children with autism. The research is still in the beginning stages, but we have seen some changes in a limited number of children by eliminating gluten and grains especially, which include improvement in GI functioning and eczema. Overall, we recommend keeping grain-based carbohydrates to a minimum and focusing more on fruits and vegetables.

Animal products

Most people are not prepared to become farmers in order to provide healthy meat options for their children. If your food budget is limited and you are not a farmer, this is where we recommend spending money for quality meat to add to your child's diet. The best quality sources for healthy meat are organic and pasture raised, which will be written on the packaging. Full-fat, pastured animal products are among the most nutritious because the fat profile has nutrients such Omega 3 and Vitamins A, E, and CLA. These have been found to be associated with a variety of health benefits (Davidson *et al.* 1999).

If you cannot find organic, pastured animal products in the grocery store, try for a local source where you can ask the farmer directly about their practices. In an ideal situation, you may be able to find a farmer who raises meats without excess exposure to chemicals and antibiotics. It is very expensive for farmers to get certified organic, so many employ organic practices but do not have official certification.

The most important concept to remember is that whatever the animal eats will be what we eat because everything they consume is stored in their meat and fat. The condition the animal has been raised in can affect its meat properties. Chronic stress and even acute stress before being slaughtered can reduce the quality of the meat product. Temple Grandin, a prominent and widely cited proponent of both animal welfare and autism rights, has made it her life's work to design animal handling systems that keep the animal from experiencing acute stress before being slaughtered for our consumption. Her extensive work and research supports the importance of humane and healthy animal treatment.

We recommend quality meat and a plant-based, wholefoods diet for children with autism. But food is not the only thing to pay attention to when thinking about diet. What your child drinks can also be helpful or problematic to their health and well-being.

Juices and sodas

This section will provide information regarding the healthiest options for drinks for children with autism and for typically developing children as well. It will provide strategies to reduce the amount of sugar found in many available children's drinks.

Most fruit juices, even organic ones, are very high in sugar. What many people do not realize is that juices possess almost the same sugar content as soda, even when freshly squeezed. When fruit is squeezed to create juice, its fiber content is eliminated and its sugar becomes concentrated. Think about how many oranges it takes to make a single glass of juice. The extracted juice is absorbed more rapidly than the whole fruit with its fiber, which can cause a surge in blood sugar and a resulting surge in insulin, triggering some inflammatory processes. I strongly encourage staying away from fruit juices and drinking water instead. If your child won't drink water, then consider watering down the juice—a little more each day until it's almost all water. You are better off from a calorie and sugar perspective with eating one orange and having a glass of water.

Even with the high sugar content of juice, there is some nutritional benefit from consumption of watered-down juices. Conversely, soda provides zero benefits for the body and also possesses many harmful properties. Many people are under the impression that diet soda is a reasonable alternative to regular soda; however, this is a misconception. Both regular and diet soda can cause an inflammatory response in the body, as well as significant weight gain, which may cause or exacerbate chronic conditions over time (Ludwig, Peterson and Gortmaker 2001; Malik, Wilett and Hu 2009; Malik *et al.* 2010). If a child is addicted to soda, do not try to reduce their intake all at once. It's best to wean the child from soda consumption on a gradual basis by beginning to add a plain seltzer to the soda to water down. Another fun option for making your own fizzled water is to purchase a home seltzer machine. I purchased an inexpensive one and have enjoyed creating different flavors of seltzer water. You can add a little natural lemon or lime for flavor; just try not to add sugar. If you really want sugar, add a little organic honey—it tastes great.

Healthy fats

Fat is an important component of a healthy diet because it helps the body build and repair itself, and it also promotes a feeling of fullness when consumed, which is very important for weight control. Of late, fats have had a bad press, one that is undeserved and unfounded according to scientific studies. When thinking about healthy and unhealthy fats, it is important to understand the different kinds of fats that can be consumed.

Just like any foods we choose to eat, fats come in a spectrum from healthy to unhealthy. They can be saturated, unsaturated, and monounsaturated. The healthiest fats are those that are monounsaturated, which are plant based. The next healthiest fats come from animals, especially those that have been pasture raised. Polyunsaturated fats are less healthy; and the least healthy are trans fats. You can refer to the ingredients label on foods to see what types of fats may be contained in the foods you are eating.

Monosaturated fats can be found in olive oil or plant-based saturated coconut oil. Olive oil is best for dressings and low temperature cooking, whereas coconut oil is perfectly suited for high temperature cooking. Other polyunsaturated oils such as nut and seed oils, corn and vegetable oils are less healthy forms of fat; they are high in Omega 6 and oxidize easily when heated. A goal to help decrease inflammation in our bodies is to increase the amount of Omega 3 we consume (fatty fish, olive oil, nuts) in relation to Omega 6, the industrial seed oils found in almost all processed foods.

There is evidence that an imbalance in the fatty acids of Omega 3 and Omega 6 may contribute to a wide range of developmental and psychiatric conditions including autism and ADHD (Richardson 2003). Trans fat, found in hydrogenated oils, is important to avoid as well. This type of fat has no known health benefits and can be detrimental to the body as it increases the amount of harmful low-density lipoprotein (LDL) cholesterol in the blood at the same time decreasing the amount of beneficial high-density lipoprotein (HDL) cholesterol. Trans fat promotes inflammation, which has been linked to heart disease, diabetes, stroke, and other chronic conditions (Mozaffarian *et al.* 2006). It's important to read labels on products that you are buying. This is actually a great lifelong skill to teach your children and especially important for a child who has autism.

TRANSLATING MENUS

This chapter has provided a wealth of information on healthy food choices, but you may be overwhelmed by the options and also be wondering how these foods can equate to a daily routine of meals. The rule of thumb is to eat mostly plant-based whole foods, but how do you translate that for your child's diet? Here is a comparison of a breakfast meal—not so healthy compared to healthier:

Sample typical breakfast:	Sample healthy breakfast:
Store brand buttermilk pancakes	· Homemade coconut pancakes (see recipe)
Store bought syrup	Maple syrup
Strawberry yogurt shake	Pastured plain Greek yogurt with berries

You may have noticed that there are no serving sizes in the examples above. This was intentional because the first place to focus is on the quality of the food, which is a more important starting point than the quantity. Food quality is all about making sure what goes into your body is helping or is neutral at best and does not cause harm. Imagine for a moment that your child's body is akin to a car. For a car to run optimally, especially if it has additional needs, you want premium gas. You want to spend a few extra dollars to prevent what could harm the engine; you don't want to end up with major repairs down the line. The same logic holds true for your child's engine. In this case, we are talking about your child's body and brain, which makes healthy eating even more important.

The science of nutrition is complex because many variables are involved at different times during digestion. Nutritional science in ASD is in its infancy, and we continue to search for links to help us better understand which elements in diet help and which might be harmful. What we know is that many children with ASD have moderate to significant GI problems and that good nutrition plays a key role in helping to support GI health. Conversely, suboptimal nutrition can do harm to GI functioning and cause children with ASD to become more susceptible to health issues, negative behaviors, and ultimately to poor long-term health outcomes.

You now have an idea of why it is important to consider what children with autism are eating. The body relies on the brain to make the best choices in feeding it. What you eat determines how well you will function on a daily basis and over time. Children with autism need every advantage under our control to help them function better, and food is one that we can regulate in order to help. The next section will provide tips for healthy cooking. After reading this information, you will be able to create your own daily recipe selection that will enable you and your family to consume healthy foods.

COOKING

The recommended diet in this book comes with one major requirement—cooking. Now before you say no way, not possible, I want you to know that cooking can be simple and quick and, dare I say, even fun, especially if you get your child involved in the preparation. It is invaluable to cultivate healthy food habits and learning for children with autism by introducing them to activities and routines that put food into a larger context that expands beyond the dinner table. Activities like grocery shopping, gardening, and cooking inspire and empower children to taste and try these foods once they sit down to eat because they have been a part of the meal creation process from the beginning. Cooking also ensures that what foods you put in your meals and ultimately in your body are helping and not harming you or your child. You are in control of all ingredients when you cook, so the bottom line is that you need to cook. It's important.

Cooking tip 1: getting organized

The best way to begin to cook is to start with the basics. Simple cooking methods help to bring out the natural flavors in foods, so it's important to remember that simple cooking can be delicious. And that's really good news for busy moms and dads. In this chapter you will find very basic cooking techniques—start simply and try more complex recipes as you gain confidence.

The key to cooking is the quality of your ingredients. Food that is in season, grown locally, and raised well tends to have the most flavor and will need the least embellishment for cooking. We promote olive oil, a little salt, and pepper, all of which compliment almost any good quality ingredient. Once you have that down, it's easy to add any kind of additional flavorings that you might like. You can pick your favorite fresh herb, which will offer a lighter seasoning than a dried herb, so you are less likely to overdo it on the seasoning.

The key is to make cooking simple and also easy so it becomes an enjoyable ritual for you and your family. Why do we like and consider potato chips as a side dish to a sandwich? Our culture likes instant gratification, and chips are quick and easy. All you have to do is open the bag and you have an instant a compliment to your main meal. The trick is to shift your thinking and practice toward making healthy foods an easy addition to your meals.

If your child really likes salad, but the thought of making salad each night seems daunting, then make the salad simple and easy. An easy suggestion is that you buy salad greens, the darker the greens, the better. Dark greens include kale, mesclun, arugula, and baby spinach, which you can buy chopped and washed at most grocery stores. Add grape tomatoes that can easily be cut in half and then some pre-shredded carrots. Toss these three foods onto a plate and voilà—you have a healthy salad!

You can prepare a week's worth of salad by getting a big colander, throwing all of your preferred ingredients into it, and thoroughly washing them with water. Divide the salad into five piles, and put each pile into a sealable Ziploc bag with a half a paper towel in each to keep the lettuce from wilting. Pull a bag out each night, and you have a fresh green salad that can be eaten as is, or you can add an extra ingredient like chicken, a little cheese, or another vegetable. You can wash out the bag and reuse it the following week to be more environmentally friendly as well.

A great tip is to take a little extra time when you get back from the grocery store to prep your own vegetables—these tend to be fresher and less expensive than buying pre-prepped vegetables. If you shop on the weekend, you can take about a half hour once you get home to wash, cut, and bag your vegetables. Then they are ready to go for any kind of cooking application during the week. You can enjoy them raw in a salad, cook them in a sauté pan, or throw them on a baking sheet for roasting.

If you incorporate a weekend food prep routine, you can avoid having to cook from scratch during the week when you're tired or get home late from work. The time-consuming part of meal prep will already be done! An added bonus is that if your kids come home starving, you can pull out your homemade ranch dressing (recipe included in the recipe section at the end of this book) and precut vegetables, and the kids will have something to nibble on while they wait for dinner. Even before you sit down to the table, the kids have already eaten their vegetables, which is another easy way to make mealtime more relaxing for everyone.

There are many cookbooks available that have healthy recipes that can be made in less than a half hour. I keep several out on my kitchen counter and use them on a regular basis. You can Google "Healthy cooking in less than an hour" and choose your favorite recipes. There are literally hundreds of recipes and resources out there, and many can be found at the back of this book!

Cooking tip 2: Learning *how* to cook

Learning to cook can be easier than you think and can also be fun, even for a busy parent. Admittedly, I was a terrible cook for many years, but I have now learned to eat healthier and to cook some really simple, yet fantastic meals. It's never too late to learn, and it's cheaper to cook in your own home than it is to buy prepared meals in the grocery store or to buy fast food. If you have very limited time, start with cooking your child's favorite foods, which may likely mean replicating fast foods like chicken nuggets and French fries. You can make a delicious and nutritious homemade version of these foods in place of the non-nutritious versions. Later in the book you will find recipes for fast food style chicken nuggets and fries that are easy to make and tasty to eat.

Did you know that you can cook food in a dishwasher? It's true! I usually begin teaching healthy cooking with a dishwasher because it's novel and fun. I cook in the dishwasher about once a week and sometimes when I need to do the dishes. I do this because it's easy and it conserves energy. The best thing about dishwasher cooking is that your children can help. It's fun and easy!

I think that dishwasher cooking is the absolute best way to poach wild caught salmon, which is an excellent source of Omega 3 fatty acids and other essential vitamins and minerals. Kids can even make their own bottled salmon just the way they like it. To do this, you will need a canning jar that seals or heavy-duty, tightly sealed aluminum foil. If you use aluminum foil for cooking, I recommend against cleaning your dishes with soap at the same time. You can put the fish and a vegetable, like broccoli or asparagus, into a canning jar with about a quarter cup of water, a few slices of lemon, and some seasoning. You can also add any other hearty vegetable that can be steamed.

Once you have your dinner in a jar, tighten the lid and place it in the upper rack of the dishwasher with your dirty dishes. Do your dishes as usual—soap and all. If the lid is fully tightened, the soap will not penetrate the jar. If you prefer not to use soap and only cook the fish and vegetables in the dishwasher, you can wrap everything in heavy-duty aluminum foil, but remember to tightly seal the aluminum foil around all edges. A number of videos that teach the art of dishwasher cooking can be found on YouTube by searching for "dishwasher cooking."

There are many other very easy recipes for healthy meals that require little effort. Another recipe I enjoy is "No peel chicken vegetable soup." It is so easy, you do not even need to peel your onion. I throw everything for chicken soup that I like in the pot. I use mostly locally-grown and organic foods: a head of broccoli, two unpeeled medium onions, four gently washed carrots (no need to peel them), and a few unpeeled, small, organic, golden potatoes.

The kids can help with this recipe, too—I have found that they usually like throwing the ingredients into the pot. Once the soup has boiled, turn down the stovetop temperature, and allow the soup to simmer over medium heat for about an hour or until the chicken is thoroughly cooked through. Once everything is cooked, you can easily pull off the onion skin, debone and scoop out the chicken, and chop up the soft vegetables. Quick, easy, healthy whole foods made simple.

See the recipes later in the book for more ideas.

TYPES OF COOKING

Cooking is broken down into two major categories—dry heat and moist heat. Dry heat cooking is when food is cooked using the temperature of the pan with an oil or fat at a higher heat for shorter periods of time. Examples of dry heat cooking are baking, roasting, and sautéing. Moist heat cooking is when food is cooked by the heat of liquid (usually water or stock) using lower temperatures for long periods of time. Types of moist heat cooking include braising, steaming, and blanching.

Dry heat cooking (baking)

Baking is the most common method of dry heat cooking and is generally done in an oven. Heat and steam are used to cook through anything from bread to meat, though baking is the most common method of dry heat cooking. Even if you don't think of yourself as a chef, you have likely used an oven, even if it was just to make boxed brownies. You can begin learning to bake by using basic ingredients to help you shift away from being dependent on pre-boxed mixes.

Baking can be as simple as following directions step by step. I recommended easing in by learning to follow a simple recipe and gradually trying more complicated recipes over time and as you build confidence. The best part about following step-by-step recipes is that your child can help. Children with autism thrive with sequenced tasks, and it's our experience that children love baking. Your meals do not need to be complicated and time consuming to be whole and nutritious. Like a muscle in the body, the more you exercise the brain through practice, the stronger you will become.

Roasting

Roasting vegetables is a mainstay in a whole foods kitchen because it's easy, and kids tend to love the flavor of roasted foods. Kids naturally shy away from many vegetables, like brussels sprouts, cauliflower, and squash; however, these can take on a remarkably sweet and pleasurable flavor when roasted. Heartier vegetables—carrots, sweet potatoes, celeriac, winter squashes, and onions—also tend to taste better when roasted.

The easiest way to roast vegetables is to cut up the vegetables into pieces—the smaller the pieces, the faster the cooking time. Place the pieces on a baking sheet in a single layer. Drizzle olive oil generously over the top, add salt and pepper, and place in a 200°C/400°F oven. Stir or flip the pieces every 10 minutes until a fork goes easily through the center.

Sautéing

Sautéing is done on the stovetop using modest heat and requires heat-stable oil like coconut, ghee, butter, or light olive oil. These oils have a higher smoke point and will not oxidize at traditional sauté temperatures. With some vegetables (woody, bitter, or with high levels of plant fiber), it may be helpful to blanch the vegetable first prior to the sautéing. Blanching instructions can be found in the next section.

Blanching

Blanching (also known as "shocking") is a great way to soften tough vegetables before dry cooking them. It is also a great way to preserve vegetables that you have too much of to eat before they go bad. Vegetables that are blanched can be bagged and frozen and will keep for about six months in the freezer.

Blanching is done by boiling water and submerging vegetables for a short period of time, usually two to four minutes, until they turn a bright color and some of their cellular structure has been softened. The vegetables are then quickly removed from the boiling water and placed in an ice bath to arrest the cooking process. The vegetables can then be cooked further for a dish or they can be bagged and frozen. When done correctly, blanching maintains important nutritional value. If vegetables begin to lose color in the boiling water, they have been overcooked and no longer have their complete nutritional value.

Braising

Braising foods is when liquid is placed at the bottom of the pan that can help steam the food while it is being baked. Braising is usually done "low and slow," meaning at a low heat over a long period of time. Braising is especially useful for tough, lower cost cuts of meat. A slow cooker, like a Crock-Pot, is ideal for these kinds of meats.

AN EATING PROGRAM FOR CHILDREN WITH SELECTIVE AND RESTRICTIVE DIETS

This section is for children who are considered picky eaters: those who may only have one to several preferred foods. This is commonly seen in many children who have autism, and parents and professionals alike find it difficult to expand the repertoire of what these children are eating.

Restricted diets

It has been well documented that many children with autism have highly selective and self-restrictive diets. Some children may only eat three or four foods during their entire childhood. Depending on what they are eating on a regular basis, this dietary habit can result in problems with nutrient and vitamin intake and potentially other more serious health problems later in life.

Children tend to fall into two camps: hypersensitive or hyposensitive eaters. Hypersensitive eaters are those with heightened sensory issues. They typically choose bland, beige foods that often are soft to eat or don't have much in terms of texture. Hyposensitive eaters are those that typically desire an additional sensory input of hard, crispy texture, and are often drawn to hyperpalatable foods like Doritos. They tend to put hot sauce on everything and like highly flavored, artificial-tasting foods. Texture aside, both groups tend to gravitate toward processed foods.

Mealtime can be a very high stress event for children with autism and their families. Many parents feel that food and nourishment are their only means of connecting with their child. The word "nourish" goes beyond just food. It is the embodiment of care and love: nurturing, healing, and whole. It is not surprising that there is a great degree of stress in homes where mealtime has historically been difficult. The majority of children with autism have feeding problems as infants. In fact, early eating difficulty may be one of the ways we begin to diagnose and get earlier intervention for children suspected of being on the autism spectrum. Rejection of food and feeding can often feel like a rejection of nurturing, which makes the entire process difficult not only for the child but for the parent or caregiver as well.

Stress and mealtime—strategies to help

The stress and anxiety that accompany mealtimes for many with autism is a huge problem. When a body is under stress, all the body's energy goes to the fight or flight response. This can then lead to a subsequent "shut down" of the GI tract (a word for what happens as a result), diminished appetite, slowed peristalsis (a word for what happens as a result), and decreased bowel activity (constipation).

These effects of stress are very important to understand because when mealtime turns stressful, there is no internal signaling for eating. Once the individual has lost this intrinsic desire for food, eating immediately becomes something that must be motivated extrinsically with things like "treat" type foods, bribery, and other outside influences. A key component of turning a child with autism into a healthy eater is to engage their intrinsic desire for food. This can be difficult, especially if mealtime has historically been a stressful event.

At The Center for Discovery, staff members Jessica Piatak, OTD, OTR/L, and Kristina Carraccia, MS, CCC-SLP, have developed a structured program to begin to get children to eat a greater variety of foods, especially foods with higher quantities of essential nutrients and vitamins. The program, called Food Exploration and Discovery (FED) Therapy, was developed for children with more severe forms of autism based on several researched methods including the works of Kay Toomey, Ph.D., Sequential Oral Sensory program; Brook Ingersoll, Ph.D., Reciprocal Imitation Training; and Marsha Dunn Klein, MEd, OTR/L, Get Permission and Trust Approach.

Often children with ASD are highly sensitive to new tastes and textures and can become very anxious if they cannot anticipate what a food will feel and taste like in their mouth. Exploration is a huge component of food acceptance. Providing experiences with food away from the table encourages exploration without causing dining room table-associated anxiety. This is why children are encouraged to tend to a garden or shop in the grocery store.

FED therapy begins slowly by introducing just one food to the child's plate or to a separate plate if they won't tolerate the food on the plate. The goal is to improve the child's relationship with food. They may not initially eat the new and nutrient-dense foods, like broccoli, but they begin to get used to seeing the food on their plate. Slowly, the child is encouraged to pick up the food, eventually bring the food to their lips, and perhaps even kiss the food. For some children, just having the food in the same room is the first step in getting them to eat a broader diet. Beginning by encouraging children to play and simply interact with the food with no pressure to consume it helps them discover how the food looks, feels, and smells.

One important point to remember is not to take away the child's preferred foods regardless of how non-nutritious without making sure that they are first accepting of new food. This process is an additive process: add the new foods before taking away the old. Children with autism can completely stop eating if you remove their preferred food in a "cold turkey" fashion. They don't seem to experience hunger like typical children. I have seen cases where children require a gastrointestinal tube to build their weight back up because preferred foods were taken away all at once. It is important to recognize that this is a slow and steady process. It takes time to broaden preferred foods. The good news is that we have been enormously successful with all of our children at The Center by following these methods.

A technique we have used with great success for children who consume highly processed foods is to substitute the same food with a mimic of that food made from scratch with higher quality ingredients. The key to mimicking McDonald's french fries is a process of twice-frying the potato with a freezing in between the frying processes. You can even initially serve them in small paper bags if that will help the child to accept the homemade version. Remember, this is a way to expand a child's food repertoire. Once these homemade fries are accepted, you can transition to oven-baked or sweet potato fries, which then become carrot or zucchini strips, and so on. I always say that once we have a green food readily accepted, we are good to go in terms of food acceptance. Green foods seem to be the hardest for most children to accept but open the most doors in terms of variety and the acceptance of healthy overall diet.

EATING AND NUTRITION REGULATION

1   4   7

Little knowledge   *Very knowledgeable*

One strategy I would like to try:

_____

Chapter 6

EMOTIONAL
SELF-REGULATION

Theresa Hamlin
with Johanna Lantz, Ph.D.

This chapter will define emotional self-regulation, and explain why this is a critical skill for a child with autism to develop. Strategies of how to teach emotional self-regulation will be provided along with techniques to develop emotional understanding. Part of the diagnosis of autism is a deficit in social and communicative skills and understanding. Emotional self-regulation is part of that deficit for many children who have more complex forms of autism.

EMOTIONAL SELF-REGULATION DEFINED

Emotional self-regulation is the ability to adjust to both negative and positive emotions based on experiences. In other words, it is having the ability to respond appropriately to the daily demands of everyday life using a range of emotions from happy to sad, nervous to calm, and angry to glad. The demands can be positive or negative, and the ability to calm and adjust to these emotions is self-regulation.

Emotional self-regulation is very complex because in order to control your emotions you need to be able to hold back, temper, and/or rev up your emotions at will. You need to control your internal body and brain states in response to a situation.

For example, you experience a situation that upsets you, such as getting a bad evaluation at work, and your brain and body will likely immediately and automatically begin to respond.

First, you may have a physiological response—a rise in your blood pressure or a quickening heartbeat. Then cognitively, your brain may go into action, thinking thoughts such as "this can't be happening," "my boss is totally off base," or "I had no idea I was perceived this way." At the same time, you may begin to feel like you have a knot in your stomach or that the hair on your neck is standing on end. Your emotional response is physical, physiological, and cognitive all at the same time. It involves multi-body systems that are highly coordinated, and yet you do this seamlessly and automatically without effort or thought.

Children with autism have great difficulty with the coordination of these systems, which causes problems with emotional self-regulation (Nader-Grosbois and Mazzone 2014). This poor self-regulation is often referred to as "dysregulation." Because of problems with their emotional system, children with autism may show increased emotional reactions to stressful events and may also have difficulty recovering once the emotional stressor has passed. The children we work with are often described as going from "zero to sixty" in a matter of seconds. In other words, one minute they appear totally calm and contented, and then seemingly out of the blue or after experiencing what seems like a minor event, they are in a full-blown emotional crisis. The children who are said to be dysregulated often rapidly shift from one emotion to another. They may perseverate (i.e., repeat a particular response) or dwell on a negative emotion or an event that caused distress and struggle to move past it. Poor emotional self-regulation interferes with thinking and learning.

JOHN

John is a 15-year-old boy with autism who was admitted into our program when a year ago he became upset and hit himself forcefully in the head. The hitting behavior caused significant swelling and bruising, which needed to be treated by his doctor. He also had quick shifts in emotion where he would go from smiling and laughing to hitting himself and crying, only to return to smiling and laughing. These shifts in emotional state all occurred within a short period of time of five minutes or less. It was difficult to determine why he was hitting himself. Sometimes he became upset when he couldn't immediately have something that he wanted, and sometimes it seemed like he became upset when he was simply asked to complete a routine task, such as taking off his shoes. There were other times when it was not clear what was bothering him. It seemed likely that there was something in the environment, possibly sensory, that he perceived as much more distressing or threatening than we did. As it turns out, he had some significant sinus problems, which most likely set the stage for the emotional overreaction. However, he was more sensitive to the environment than most of his peers.

CHILDREN WITH AUTISM AND EMOTIONAL SELF-REGULATION

Researchers have studied differences in emotional self-regulation between children with autism and their peers without autism. Samson, Huber, and Gross (2012) found that people with autism reported more negative emotions than people without autism, but both groups reported equal amounts of positive emotions. They also discovered that people with autism had more difficulty understanding and explaining their own emotions and also were less likely to use coping strategies or strategies to help them calm down, such as cognitive reappraisal (i.e. reshaping how you think about certain situations).

Emotional dysregulation can occur when children with autism are overwhelmed by their sensory environment. Green *et al.* (2013) were interested in the brain's response to mildly aversive sounds and images in individuals with autism and those without autism. Using fMRI brain imaging technology, they found that the children with autism showed greater activation in their brains when exposed to mildly aversive stimuli, demonstrating that the mildly aversive sounds or images negatively affected them more than their peers who did not have autism. In previous chapters, I presented ways in which people with autism respond differently behaviorally and at the biological level to perceived stress in the environment. We can learn from these studies to broaden our understanding about why children demonstrate negative reactions to seemingly benign events.

GARRET

In 2013, a family brought their nine-year-old son, Garret, to us for a three-day evaluation. Their trip included a two-hour wait in the airport for the plane, a three-hour plane ride, and a two-hour car ride before reaching our Bed and Breakfast. Despite the grueling seven-hour trip, the young boy arrived and entered the B&B with high energy, darting from corner to corner of the living room. His emotional state was in high gear. He was immediately drawn to the vacuum cleaner that was left out in the corner of the room and began flipping the cord to the vacuum. His dad, who looked like he had traveled a full 24 hours without sleep, commented that his son loves cords and will self-stimulate or "stim" on them for hours when he's in a new place.

During the three-day stay, each time Garret was brought to a new space, he would dart around the room looking for a cord or something similar to flip. After he had been allowed time to adjust to the new spaces by flipping a familiar object, he was able to engage in an activity, and his emotional state became obviously calmer. This behavior of flipping, although seemingly without purpose, calmed Garret down so that he could engage in the new and unfamiliar environment. The behavior appeared to serve a self-regulating function.

It's important to take notice of these types of behaviors. If they are not all consuming or do not overly interfere with daily functioning, you can use an additive approach: rather than targeting these behaviors for elimination, begin instead with adding another positive strategy. In this case, the child was taught to use a schedule. This began to organize his experiences, which helped regulate his emotional state. Over time, it is very likely that the flipping behavior will diminish as his emotional response system becomes more regulated.

PSYCHOLOGICAL STRESS

Stress is a factor in everyone's lives, but too much stress or chronic stress can jeopardize one's well-being. The contribution of stress to the behaviors and overall health of children with autism is often not recognized or considered when developing treatment. This is unfortunate given the connection between stress and the ability to self-regulate. This section describes the potentially harmful effects of stress and the importance of predictability and control in moderating the effects of stress.

Sapolsky (2004), a leading authority on emotional regulation and stress, and other researchers (Glaser and Kiecolt-Glaser 2005), have demonstrated that psychological stress can activate the body's stress response chronically enough to create disease consequences in the body. When children with autism are chronically anxious and stressed by complex social settings or new and unpredictable settings/events, their emotions and thoughts can make them sick. Sapolsky noted that you are more vulnerable to stress if the following are true:

* You lack social support or perceive that you are alone.

* You feel that you don't have options in a bad situation.

* You're not getting any predictive information—in other words, you don't know how bad things might get or when they might end.

* You feel like you have no control.

* You interpret things as getting worse.

Hans Selye (1936) first identified evidence of stress-related diseases in humans. According to Seyle there were a wide array of stressors that could cause pathologies or problems in the body and mind. As you learned in the first set of chapters, when the body is subjected to prolonged stressors, the stress response over time will do damage to the body's health. Some of the common repercussions of chronic stress include obesity, malabsorption problems, GI problems, immune disorders, ulcers, impaired reproduction, and other chronic diseases (Purdy 2013). From a health perspective, over activation of the stress response in the long run can be very problematic.

In a series of studies, Glass and Singer (1972a) suggested that stress would result in adverse effects only when it disrupts an individual's ability to feel that their experience is inadequately organized and when it threatens their belief in or view of themselves as being able to organize their experience. In other words, you have to perceive the threat. If you have a "happy go lucky" personality, you're going to experience less of a stress response and effect even if your world is falling apart around you. Researchers emphasize that unpredictable aversive events achieve a stress-arousing effect because the individual believes that they cannot control the onset and/or offset of the event. There is a perception of helplessness at the center of the stress reaction.

Psychological stress can be reduced when the child feels in control and when the stress is predictable. Even when a stressful event occurs, if it occurs with a high degree of predictability then it is less stressful on the body. Predictability and control over the environment and stressful events are very important factors in reducing stress. For example if your child finds getting on the school bus each morning to be stressful, it actually is less stressful than it could be if it didn't occur every day. If the school bus arrived on a random schedule and not every day at 7:30am, this would be much more stressful for them. Not knowing is really worse than knowing. The good news is that the stress that occurs during these situations can be reduced by teaching the child how to self-calm their body and mind. It may not always stop the initiation of the autonomic stress response, but it can lessen the length and degree of the response.

In summary, children with autism often have difficulty regulating their emotions, which can lead to maladaptive behaviors, social difficulties and psychological distress. The chronic and extreme stress experienced by those with autism who struggle to make sense of the world further impacts day-to-day functioning. The remainder of this chapter will describe techniques to help build self-regulation and decrease stress.

TECHNIQUES FOR GAINING CONTROL OF THE ENVIRONMENT

Sapolsky's (2004) extensive research has taught us that gaining control of the environment is an excellent way to reduce stress and increase regulation. Many children with autism, particularly those who are more severely affected, have skill deficits that limit their independence. Therefore, they have less opportunity to exert control over what is happening in their own lives. A sense of helplessness can develop that extends beyond environmental control to self-control. Feelings of helplessness can lead to anxiety and mood disorders. This section offers techniques to give children more control over their lives including functional communication training (FCT), offering choices, increasing predictability, and gaining control of the sensory environment.

Functional communication training

Functional communication training (FCT) is an approach where children are taught how to communicate basic wants and needs. The form of communication varies and is based on the child's skills. Communication can include verbal responses, picture exchange, voice output technology, or gestures.

For those who are more severely affected by autism, it is important to evaluate the extent to which they can communicate basic wants and needs. Imagine how frustrated you would feel if you had to spend even one day without being able to communicate with others. I know that I would feel I had little control over what was happening in my life and would likely grab someone by the shoulders or face to get their attention just to try to feel like I was in control once again. Giving someone who cannot communicate the ability to do so gives them the chance to take control, which helps reduce frustration and increase self-regulation. When children do not have the ability to communicate effectively, they often have no other choice but to resort to using problem behaviors to get their needs met.

Functional communication training usually starts with a functional behavioral assessment (FBA) to determine whether the child is attempting to communicate through maladaptive or inappropriate behaviors. In school settings, the FBA is typically completed by a school psychologist. If you feel you understand what your child desires to communicate, FCT can also be done without an FBA. For example, in functional communication training, a child who becomes upset when a task becomes too challenging learns to ask for a break or for help instead. A child who becomes socially overwhelmed is taught to request time alone. Sometimes, it may be necessary to teach children to ask for attention from others or just to ask for things they want.

Teaching functional communication can be done by designing situations where the child is motivated to communicate. For example, if you want to teach the child how to ask for help, you can give them a container with a preferred item inside that they cannot open and provide a prompt to request help. To teach children to request attention, you would prompt them to tap someone on the shoulder, raise their hand, or call someone by name. At the same time, you would ignore other maladaptive behaviors that are typically used to gain attention. To teach asking for time alone, you would identify a situation in which a child typically appears overwhelmed and prompt them to communicate that they need to be away from others. Following successful communication, even if prompted, you would escort the child to a quiet location.

All prompts used during teaching are gradually phased out. When teaching new skills, it is best to start with the most prompting needed such as a physical prompt and then fade back to just a verbal prompt and then no prompt. This is referred to as "errorless" learning because it ensures that the child is responding correctly most of the time, which is important for self-efficacy and motivation. Repetition is also important. Once a communication target is chosen, the child should have the opportunity to practice several times per day to gain the skill more quickly. Furthermore, they should practice with multiple people in multiple settings in order for the communication skill to be generalized to other people and places.

Offering choices

Another way to increase control over the temporal environment is to allow your child to make choices in their day. Choices should be simple; two are usually sufficient because more may overwhelm the child. For example, ask your child to choose either a green or blue marker, or choose whether to brush their teeth now or in five minutes. Choices allow your child to have a say in what they want to do instead of always being told what to do by others. This is empowering and can boost self-efficacy and engagement with the environment.

Increasing predictability of environment

As described above, a more predictable environment helps to alleviate stress. One of the best ways to make the environment more predictable is through use of written or picture schedules. This is especially important when there is a change to the normal routine. You can also incorporate choice into schedules by allowing places in the schedule where the child is allowed to choose the activity. Priming is a memory effect in which exposure to one situation influences a response to another situation. It is a way to prepare children for what to do in novel situations. Priming can include reading a social story or showing a video of what the person will be expected to do and what objects and people will likely be present prior to engaging in a new or potentially stressful situation. More ideas for increasing predictability of the environment through visual and physical supports were provided in Chapter 4.

The following is an example of how increasing the predictability of a child's day through the use of schedule helped decrease his stress levels.

DAVID

David, like many children we see who have autism, becomes highly stressed whenever there is an unpredictable event such as an unexpected change to the schedule or staffing in the classroom. When he goes home at night, his mother reports similar problems when their schedule changes or when a home aide doesn't come for a particular reason. The stress is evident by his high EDA response and loss of ability to focus on whatever the event is, and there is usually an aggressive behavior such as hitting or slapping. In order to decrease his stress response, we have given him more predictability by creating a visual schedule of all staff and/or students who come and go during the day and evening, and any possible substitutes that may occur when a scheduled activity is cancelled. The schedule is a predictable schedule of the unpredictable daily events. David reviews the schedule several times each day and at least twice at night so he can see possible substitutions before an unpredictable event occurs. When he has this schedule, he is less likely to exhibit a stress response because at least he knows that people will come and go unpredictably during the day and that schedule changes may happen. Knowing is better than not knowing and being taken by surprise. He has also been taught to request a rest time, a walk, and/or to deep breathe if he is becoming stressed. Thus, he is learning to self-calm and self-regulate when he becomes upset.

Control over the sensory environment

Children with ASD can be sensitive to sensory stimuli. They may be sensory seeking or trying to avoid situations. Those who seek to avoid may engage in behaviors to reduce exposure such as covering their ears or eyes or crawling under blankets or pillows. Those who are sensory seeking may engage in constant movement or look for other forms of input from the environment such as banging on objects or pressing their chin on others. When the sensory environment becomes overwhelming, a variety of responses can occur. Some children may desire to escape the situation; some children may show an increase of motor activity or agitation; some children may shut down. The sensory environment can interfere with the child's ability to self-regulate. Although all senses can be impacted in autism, we have found that noise affecting the auditory sensory system is particularly problematic because it is often very difficult to control in the classroom and community.

Many researchers have examined the impact of noise on people. Noise has been found to increase aggression in people who are already aroused, upset, or angry (Donnerstein and Wilson 1976). Researchers have also discovered that allowing people to have control over noise reduces the probability of aggressive behavior (Geen 1978) and improves task performance (Glass and Singer 1972b). Furthermore, people exposed to uncontrollable noise have been shown to experience greater levels of physiological arousal, such as higher blood pressure and pulse, compared to those who could control the noise (Geen and McCown 1984). The bottom line is that giving people the option to control noise helps to reduce the stress associated with noise.

This idea is evident in the instance of Calvin, who was very sensitive to noises in his environment.

CALVIN

Calvin, who was also mentioned in Chapter 3, experienced distress when he heard the vocalizations of particular peers who are in his class. The vocalizations were recorded on an iPad and Calvin listened to the recordings. At first he was taught to turn off the recording. The idea that he could have control over the sound at least part of the time worked to decrease his stress levels upon hearing the vocalizations. After he was able to do this successfully, we taught him to request "I want quiet" by using a voice output program on his iPad. Following the request for quiet, Calvin was allowed to put on noise-cancelling headphones for five minutes. Putting on noise-cancelling headphones allowed Calvin to dampen the noise while still remaining in the classroom. This intervention utilized both noise control and functional communication training. Calvin had control of the situation because he now had a way to communicate when he needed quiet and then was able to take a break from the noise using the headphones.

To conclude, providing children with autism with a means to gain better control over their environment is an important way to reduce stress. These techniques are based in best practices and can be used in home and on demand for a child who is experiencing stress. The following section explains a number of additional techniques that not only can be used for children with autism, but by most people as we all experience stress in our lives.

TECHNIQUES TO REDUCE STRESS AND PROMOTE RELAXATION

With mounting evidence that emotional awareness and emotional regulation promote healthy minds, bodies, and relationships, it's important to find ways to help children with autism understand and positively influence their emotions. The good news is that we can do something about stress! Children with autism, as well as their caregivers, can learn to use stress reduction strategies when the feeling of stress arises. This section lists techniques that have been proven to work for children with autism, including progressive muscle relaxation, music therapy, mindfulness, yoga, and more.

Progressive muscle relaxation

Progressive muscle relaxation is a sequenced relaxation technique of all muscle groups from head to toe. It is not only good for relaxation but also for overall body awareness. The progression begins with the head and neck, moves to the arms, belly, buttocks, and legs, and ends with the feet and toes. The slow and thoughtful process keeps the attention focused on your breathing as well as the large muscle of the body. Once practiced, the person experiences a calmer, more relaxed state.

In some variations of this technique, the person leading the relaxation uses imagery such as squeezing lemons or pretending a fly is landing on your muscle to prompt you to tighten a particular muscle. While many children with less severe forms of autism can follow this imagery, other children struggle to use their imagination and are therefore less successful at following more abstract directions.

Cautela and Groden (1978) developed a program to teach progressive muscle relaxation to children with autism and other related disabilities that can be found in their book *Relaxation: A Comprehensive Manual for Adults, Children and Children with Special Needs*. This technique has been adapted by occupational therapists at The Center for Discovery, using various props to help make the tasks more concrete, to assist with motor planning and coordination, and to deliver in either in a group or individual format. An adaptation might be a hula-hoop with foam attachments, which is used for students to squeeze and release, or a Bosu ball that is placed under the table for the students to press their feet against the ball and release. Parents, teachers, and therapists can guide children using progressive muscle relaxation techniques. It is easily be done anywhere, and it's sequential and orderly—all positives for success for a child with autism.

Music therapy

It has been said by many that music is a universal language. Children of all ages and abilities seem to enjoy music. Several studies have been conducted using music to teach emotional and self-regulation to children (Moore 2013). Music therapy has also has been found to reduce stress and anxiety in children with autism (Hillier *et al.* 2011; Kim, Wigram and Gold 2009). We have been using music therapy in the form of intensive therapy, where a child receives music therapy for one hour, four to five times per week for a duration of eight to ten weeks. Our results have demonstrated that the children become more relaxed, attentive, and focused as the sessions progress from week to week. The increased attention and decreased perceived stress has been documented to extend into the classroom post the therapy session.

A music therapy technique

Drumming at 60 beats per minute can be used to soothe children who are experiencing high amounts of stress. Drumming has been very successful in increasing focused attention and appropriate responding. If you don't have access to a music therapy program, I would advise going online and looking for 60-beat drum music. My favorite is "60 BPM—simple straight beat—drum track," which can be played on a drum beat metronome and seems to help reduce stress. You can control the beat by either increasing or decreasing the beat right online. Your child can very easily manipulate this program and use it as a calming technique. Mealtime is a good time to experiment with the drumbeat in the background, as digestion could be aided by the beat. Don't be concerned if your child begins to rock with the music—it will aid in calming their whole body. I regularly find myself slightly rocking or at least tapping my feet to the beat.

Mindfulness

Practicing mindfulness is also a very good way to reduce stress, as it focuses your attention on the present. Through this technique, the child learns to control their emotional state. Mindfulness is about learning to be present, to listen, and to observe in the moment. It teaches you to keep your mind on what is happening in the immediate environment versus allowing the mind to wander during interactions. Learning to be mindful takes practice, but it can really make a difference when combating stress.

Rechtschaffen (2014), an authority on mindfulness, has guided our initial work on mindfulness at The Center for

Discovery. To begin to teach mindfulness, he uses a fruit like an orange as a tool to teach the concept of being present. He asks the children and adults to first hold and view the orange in their hands for several minutes while focusing on all the details that would describe the orange—shape, color, size, texture, how it reflects light, and so on. Then, the audience smells the orange and describes the smell. This is followed by a deliberately slow peeling of the orange. Once the orange is peeled, attention returns to the color and texture of the new form that the orange takes. After another minute of exploration, the participants take five unhurried minutes to taste and ultimately eat the orange. A discussion then follows about how the child or adult felt about their level of focus, first talking about the orange, but then generalizing to daily encounters.

MindUp, sponsored by the Hawn Foundation (2011), is an evidence-based and commercially available curriculum that offers lessons in mindfulness and includes enjoyable activities that make the abstract concept of mindfulness more understandable.[1] Each lesson provides concrete information on how the brain functions while attending. It is presented in language easily understood by children of varying age groups. The students explore the topics by engaging in hands-on activities. It includes what is called "Core Practice" that is meant to be done two to four times per day. "Core Practice" is a guided practice in deep belly breathing and attentive listening. MindUp is appropriate for students with less severe forms of ASD.

Try it!

In order to teach mindfulness to children, it may helpful for you to understand what it feels like for yourself. Begin by identifying just one activity you will be mindful with. For example, you might try practicing mindfulness while eating a snack at work or home.

---

1   See http://thehawnfoundation.org/mindup/

Let's practice. Even if you only have a piece of lettuce or a raisin on hand start with that. First, look carefully at what you are going to be eating. Examine the color, size, texture, and the minute details of the food. Slow down; take note of each feature. Before you take your first bite, smell the food and notice if your mouth salivates. Take your first bite and focus on the taste of the food as you move it around in your mouth. Keep the food in your mouth; chew it slowly and thoroughly. Swallow slowly so that you can feel the food traveling down the esophagus to the stomach. Repeat the process one more time. Now, take a moment to reflect on the process. You may feel a sense of calmness, if only for a moment. If you don't, do not worry. Mindfulness practice is called practice for a reason. When practiced regularly, you will hopefully begin to experience a heightened sense of awareness and calm. The idea is that you will eventually be able to summon the feeling from experience when you are experiencing heightened stress.

The next section offers a technique that combines movement with awareness and mindfulness practice: yoga.

Yoga

Yoga is a systematic practice of exercise that builds body strength and flexibility. The breathing taught through the practice helps calm the mind as the child is taught to focus on their breath. Yoga is known to lower blood pressure, slow the heart rate, and has been demonstrated to lower cholesterol and triglyceride levels while increasing immune functioning (Chu *et al.* 2014). The therapeutic effects of yoga can increase quality of life (Woodyard 2011).

Yoga can also help with balance and with problems in the cerebellum, two issues that have been noted in children with autism (Betts and Betts 2006). Balance poses, especially those requiring a child to support themselves on one foot, can be helpful for improving attention and cerebellum functioning. The balance poses demand full attention and focus from second to second or you lose the pose. Thoughts and emotions are also brought into balance as our efforts are focused on maintaining a pose. The simple act of balancing can bring calmness and promote self-control.

Children with autism that participated a school-based yoga program called "Get Ready to Learn" were studied for 16 weeks. It was discovered that the students in the program demonstrated a significant decrease in maladaptive behavior when compared to the students who were not in the program (Koenig, Buckley-Reen and Garg 2012).

Yoga can also be fun for children with autism. Teaching yoga poses by demonstrating the pose, paired with actual photos of the pose, is a good way to begin to help children see and experience how to practice yoga. A series of six or seven poses is sufficient for a child to develop a nice routine that can be practiced daily.

Vigorous exercise break

Teaching the child to request a time out for a vigorous exercise break is a very successful intervention technique that we use for calming the mind and body. If the child cannot yet request time out, then simply building in time for vigorous exercise throughout the day can be very helpful to them. In Chapter 7 on energy regulation there are many examples and "how tos" of quick exercises such as jumping jacks or burpees that can be incorporated throughout the day. Hand in hand with exercise comes learning to take calming breaths. The next section will teach how to incorporate breathing into a child's daily routine.

Meditation and breath

In addition to mindfulness practice and yoga, deep breathing is a helpfulness technique for reducing stress. Deep breathing imposes a rhythm on the autonomic nervous system and restores order to the body and mind. It counteracts cortisol, slows your heart rate, and brings increased CO_2 (Carbon Dioxide) into the blood. Decreased CO_2 in the blood can be triggered by shallow, fast breathing when stressed, which promotes feelings of anxiety and fear. These feelings can then trigger the fight or flight reaction in the body. A person needs a healthy balance between oxygen and carbon dioxide in their blood. Restoring carbon dioxide through deep breathing is a way to reverse the stress cycle. When practiced daily, it is one of the most powerful and useful tools we have to maintain a calm state, decrease anxiety, and recover from stress—it's free and readily available today.

Deep breathing: let's try it!

Find a comfortable place to sit, and keep your back straight. It is preferable to cross your legs, but you can sit on a chair instead. The important thing is to be comfortable. You do not need to add more stress than you are already experiencing. Keep your shoulders relaxed and down (as opposed to hunched up close to your neck, which is a common response to stress). Keep your eyes open or closed, whichever you prefer. If you keep your eyes open, focus on an object nearby to avoid distractions. Place your hands palms up or down on the tops of your knees. Move one hand to your chest and the other hand on your belly. Take a very deep, long breath in through nose to the count of eight. Try to envision the air coming in as the color blue. With your hand on your belly, feel your stomach rising and expanding as it fills with air. Hold the inhalation for five seconds and then begin to release the air slowly through your mouth to count of eight. Try to see the air being released as red. With your other hand on your chest, feel your chest falling as air is released. Repeat this breathing exercised five times or more if needed. As this breathing techniques gets easier, you can alternate the practice. You may prefer to keep your hands on your knees at all times or by your side.

There is a Breathing Lessons app that can be purchased through iTunes that is an excellent tool to teach guided deep breathing, or you can practice and teach yourself without the app. There is also a free app called Stop, Breathe & Think. It gives you suggestions for how long to meditate based on your response to emotions from the day.

Nature connection

Nature should not be overlooked as a method to reduce stress. Just seeing greenery can reduce stress in people. Spending time in nature and the great outdoors can be a powerful tool to help a child regulate their emotions, especially when they are in a stressful situation. The increasing complexity of our fast-paced world, with its dependence on technology and closed, indoor environments to live, learn, and work, can be a source of stress especially if there is little time to go outside. Conversely, the nurturing properties of the green natural environment can help to ameliorate stress and provide maintenance for health and well-being. The remedy for those living in a high-paced, highly dense urban area is spending time in natural areas. Typically people living in urban environments choose to take a trip to the beach, a walk in the park, or drive through the country to get away from the stress of urban living. These are the types of settings that we intuitively know help reduce stress. Nature is restorative, and our bodies and mind can feel this. If you live in a rural area, then you already have a natural relaxing platform.

Ulrich and colleagues (Ulrich *et al.* 1991) measured people's response to viewing outdoor nature scenes on videos versus viewing urban scenes on video such as buildings, traffic on streets, and general street scenes. In a controlled experiment, he and his colleagues first exposed everyone in the study to an emotionally stressful video of the horrors of work accidents. Then, they randomly divided the group into two, showing short videos of nature scenes to one group and short videos of urban scenes to the other group. The researchers found that in all cases there was a positive restoration of the body to a resting state, as measured by physiological functions including skin conductance, blood pressure, heart rate, and tension of the frontalis muscle of the forehead. The resting state, however, occurred more rapidly and was more complete for people viewing the nature scenes versus the urban scenes. The people viewing nature were more relaxed. In other words, when people are given the choice between scenes that contain nature versus scenes without nature, nature almost always wins out.

In another experiment, Ulrich (1984), who was interested in the effects of nature on stress and healing, studied patients who had undergone a surgical procedure. He compared the recovery rates for those recuperating who had a window view of trees versus those who had a window view of bricks and mortar. The former recuperated faster than those without a nature view. Additionally, the patients with the nature view required less use of pain management medication, showed increased pleasantness toward the nurses, and spent fewer days in the hospital. These positive repercussions resulted in a reduction in overall medical costs. Ulrich's work helped expand our understanding of nature as it relates to human health and healing, including how the body and the brain are affected by nature.

At The Center, we have found that when a child with autism is stressed, upset, or frustrated, they will almost always calm down when brought into nature. The same holds true for the staff interacting with the child.

When immediate access to a natural or outdoor space that has green vegetation is not available, showing short videos of nature scenes is a backup option for regulating the emotional system. According to Ulrich *et al.* (1991), our bodies and our minds have been biologically prepared to respond to landscapes that helped set our physiological and psychological patterns. Seeing green nature and participating in activities that are nature based, like gardening or playing in the grass, enhances our well-being. Even if you're living in an urban environment, you can still create micro-restorative green spaces that can be extremely beneficial for stress reduction and emotional regulation. Rooftop or windowsill gardens are a great way to start. There are many house plants that do very well inside and require little attention beyond watering; they also have the added benefit of improving the indoor air quality. Green vegetation makes a positive difference to our psychological state.

TECHNIQUES TO DEVELOP EMOTIONAL UNDERSTANDING

Another key element of emotional regulation is learning to understand one's own thoughts and feelings and the feelings of others. Teaching basic mood awareness and recognition of feelings is especially helpful for those individuals who have mood disorders or difficulty understanding others' feelings. Furthermore, emotional understanding is critical to the development of social relationships. This section will introduce techniques and therapies meant to help children with autism better understand their emotions and those of others.

Cognitive behavioral therapy (CBT)

One technique for developing emotional understanding is called cognitive behavioral therapy, also known as CBT. CBT is an evidence-based therapy that is highly effective for treating mood and anxiety disorders in the general population (Lang *et al.* 2010b). Brain imaging studies have shown that CBT can produce changes similar to medication at the neurological level (Goldapple *et al.* 2004).

Participants in this type of therapy are taught to be observant of what they are thinking about in a particular situation. Then they are taught to think about how those thoughts make them feel and how thoughts and feelings lead to reactions and behaviors. Behavior change can occur when children begin to change the way they think about a situation or event.

CBT calls for approaches such as exposure to situations that cause anxiety such as a child calling on a classmate in front of their peers when they have social anxiety, or going to a park with grassy areas when they have a fear of bees. CBT also includes exercises that challenge the beliefs that are distorted or irrational. There is a growing body of research that shows that modified CBT treatments are effective for those with less severe forms of ASD who also suffer from anxiety (Storch *et al.* 2015; Wood *et al.* 2009). Wood and colleagues (Wood *et al.* 2015) developed a CBT treatment program specifically for those with autism called *Behavioral Interventions for Anxiety in Children with Autism* or BIACA. This program includes modifications to more traditional CBT programs such as incorporating the child's special interests into therapy. It is important to find a clinician with expertise in CBT and also ASD. There are an increasing number of providers who are able to provide this therapy. A good resource for finding a provider is available at the Association for Behavioral and Cognitive Therapies website.[2]

Cognitive reappraisal is one primary component of CBT. Cognitive reappraisal is an emotional regulation strategy that involves changing the trajectory of an emotional response. It is essential to first recognize that you are having an emotional response and then be able to reinterpret the situation to reduce the severity of the response, or change the response to a positive one. Timing is crucial, as you do not want to give the negative thought too much time to settle in. It is important for parents and teachers to help the child recognize the negative emotion; label it (I'm mad, frustrated, feeling helpless...); then find a positive substitution using techniques such as constructed

---

2   http://abctcentral.org

empathy (seeing oneself in another's shoes), it could be worse, or visualize the best case scenario. For example, if a child becomes upset because they have to wait for his sister to put on her shoes before they can leave to go to dinner, the child can express that they are "mad" or "frustrated" either in words or by pointing to a picture that reflects that emotion. This verbal or visual expression is taught in lieu of hitting someone or having a temper tantrum. The child can then be prompted to express how that situation could be worse, such as the sister not only needing to put on her shoes, but also needing to take a shower first. This simple comparison can help put the situation into perspective: it could be worse. This technique can help the child to calm down. If the child does not yet have the cognitive ability to do this type of reappraisal thinking, then showing them a picture of the emotion and stating that you understand they are upset, and then using a count-down strip, can sometimes help to relieve the frustration and stress that the child is experiencing.

When you apply reappraisal techniques, your body and brain will not respond with the same level of reactive "fight or flight" stress response because your higher order thinking process takes control of the situation. You change your brain's perception of the event. This technique can be used to help children who have autism. When the perceived stressful event or situation arises in real time, quickly apply the reappraisal strategy. Heather L. Urry (2010) noted that it takes ten seconds for a positive thought to be held in your mind in order to replace the negative response. This takes practice, but for many children who have the cognitive ability to think about, identify, and articulate their emotions, it's a good strategy.

As an example, I was driving home the other night on a long and windy country road. About three miles from my home, I got stuck behind a driver who was traveling at about the speed of a snail. Because the road was narrow with many blind curves, I couldn't really pass him. I could see it was an older driver, and I could also feel a sense of frustration brewing inside of me very quickly. I was tired, had to cook dinner, walk the dogs, attend an online class, help my son pack for a trip, and so on. I had a lot to do, and every minute mattered to me. However, there was nothing I could do to get around this driver.

Having spent so much time studying emotional regulation, I figured I should put it to use. I was able to talk myself out of frustration by using a cognitive reappraisal technique. That is, I thought about how the situation could be worse, reappraising it.

I thought about the fact that I could have been behind this driver for my full ten miles of back roads and not just two short miles. I also thought that this older gentleman could be like my grandfather, probably had difficulty seeing and hearing very well, and I wouldn't want to frighten him by passing his car or blowing my horn. I was able to calm myself down by thinking that it could have been worse and by trying to empathize with the older driver using the "other shoe" or constructed empathy technique. I turned up the (slow tempo) music in my car, and enjoyed the ride at a snail's pace. In the end, I was actually more focused when I got home. It's amazing all the things you see when you slow down.

The Incredible 5-Point Scale

There are many commercially available programs designed to help children with ASD develop better emotional understanding and self-regulation that incorporate components of CBT. These programs capitalize on the visual strengths of those with ASD and their desire for order and cause and effect relationships. One such program was created by Dunn-Buron and Curtis (2012) and is referred to as The Incredible 5-Point Scale. This program aligns thoughts, feelings, and behaviors on a five-point scale. For example, a scale may be developed for a child that describes what they look like and feel like at a "five" when then are angry, a "four" when they are less angry, and so on. This is then tied with positive social strategies they can use at each number. At a five on the scale, the child may indicate that they are throwing books and screaming that they feel like they are going to explode, and that they need to leave the area and take a walk instead. The paired strategy that they might use when at this level of stress would be to leave the area, go outside for fresh air, if possible, and engage in a ten-minute bout of vigorous exercise.

Zones of regulation

Another great commercially available, social-emotional curriculum is the Zones of Regulation (Kuypers 2011) program. The Zones curriculum includes a workbook and CD with activities. The curriculum incorporates aspects of the Incredible 5-Point Scale, as well as Williams and Shellenberger (1996) Alert program.

Zones aims to teach self-regulation and emotional control. There are four zones: red, yellow, green, and blue. The red zone is when the student feels out of control. The yellow zone is when the student is experiencing some distress but is still in control. The green zone is when the student is happy and focused. The blue zone is when the student is experiencing low levels of arousal and alertness. Students learn to recognize what zone they are in and to use a "tool box" of cognitive, sensory, and calming strategies to self-regulate. Problem solving, emotional recognition, and perspective taking are also taught through various activities that are part of the curriculum. These skills are important for emotional regulation as they increase the child's ability to understand the thoughts and feelings of other people. Confusion about what others are thinking and feeling can cause emotional distress and also makes it difficult to form social relationships.

Identifying feelings

In addition to these programs, there are several ways to build self-regulation that are easily implemented without a formal program. Some techniques use pictures of situations and accompanying feeling lists. The child chooses from a list of feelings the one that best matches the situation in the picture and then actually feels or "tries on" the particular emotion. The child may then use a mirror to view their reflection and see if their image matches that of the picture image. The goal is for the child to become increasingly aware of how emotions look and feel so they may ultimately become aware of their own emotional state and body language—facial expression, breathing, and body tensions—as measures of stress or calmness. This is a great activity to do before bed. It requires focus and can end with finding the picture that matches a calm self, which is an important component of a healthy bedtime routine.

Stories and videos

Stories and videos can be used to teach children with autism better understand emotions. Stories that children watch in movie form or read in books can be used to raise awareness of fear or other strong emotions that children may naturally experience without realizing it. Once brought into consciousness in a relaxed setting, they can then be discussed without triggering an actual stress response. The frontal lobe controls the higher order thinking part of the brain and is active during a controlled and conscious situation, whereas the emotional part of the brain is in the limbic system, which is reactive, instinctive and automatic during perceived stress events. When children are able to take the time to think reasonably about a particular fear or stress event, and reattribute or reappraise it, then it can have less of a debilitating effect.

While watching a movie or reading a book, you can stop the movie or story and talk about why the character is acting in a certain way. This discussion can then lead into talking about similar situations that the child may experience and can help to shape how they react in those instances. For example, if you are watching a pre-recorded sitcom and one character begins to raise their voice at another character in frustration, you can discuss times when the child may have been very frustrated and also felt like yelling or did yell. Then you can talk about a healthier way to handle the situation from a third party perspective.

Every evening presents a new opportunity to find a story that has an example of what not to do when you're stressed; conversely, many of these TV programs will also portray more positive and healthy ways of handling situations. This exercise is a great way to make watching TV instructive and interactive. I also recommend acting out the drama, if appropriate, which is a great strategy for supporting long-term memory and recall of the situation.

Another fun activity is to have your child watch a television show without the sound. You then discuss what the characters are feeling and how they may be expressing their emotions. This exercise works on understanding nonverbal behaviors that give us clues about the emotional states of others. For beginners, the *Candid Camera* show is a good choice. It highlights basic emotions, such as surprise, anger, and happiness. It is also helpful for working on Theory of Mind, which is described in the section below entitled "Techniques to foster empathy." *Candid Camera* is available through online retailers.

If your child has not yet developed the social or cognitive skills needed to recognize and discuss emotions being viewed, then you can use pictures of faces that can be paired with emotions. Dramatically depicted emotions on faces are the best. You can cut out 8" x 10" size pictures of faces that represent various emotions and glue them to a tongue depressor, and even laminate for durability. You just need to Google pictures of emotions and you have a wide variety to choose from. A good set of dramatic pictures of emotions can also be found online by entering a search for pictures of emotions.[3] When watching TV or reading a story with your child, you can ask them to choose the picture that bests matches the emotion being viewed. You can also model the emotion by choosing the correct picture yourself, and then have your child choose the emotion. Always label the emotion by saying what it is: happy, sad, scared, or confused, and so on. I also recommend incorporating a mirror so that the child can not only pick a picture of the emotion, but also try the emotion on and see it expressed on their face by looking in the mirror. Once your child becomes acquainted with the various emotions, you can begin to use them during real life situations. Try not to over complicate the emotions; just choose a few of the most common ones to begin.

Write about it

There is a lot that we can do to change how we think and perform under pressure. Children with autism can freeze or "melt down" under stressful conditions. In their 2011 research study of high schoolers, Rameriz and Beilock demonstrated that a simple writing exercise performed before a test could reduce anxiety enough that those who engaged in the writing outperformed their peers by more than half a letter grade. Beilock has continued by looking at the internal mechanisms of the anxious brain to see how it changes during stressful situations. It appears that writing about your emotions, for example, "I get really nervous during tests, my hands sweat, and I get confused even though I know the information…" can be very effective in breaking the negative cycle of thinking. Beilock has said that the stress is like having too many computer programs open in your brain at one time, and that writing helps to shut some of them down, allowing a person to think more clearly.

----

3   www.wikihow.com

Although the use of writing to alleviate stress has not been trialed on children with autism, it seems plausible that it could be effective because stress is a universal phenomenon. Some children with autism enjoy writing and may do so repetitively. This technique may be particularly helpful for those with this profile. Emotional writing was born out of the science of writing to combat depression and trauma, which has been used quite successfully to decrease worrying. A social story that uses words or pictures may be trialed for children who are not able to engage in writing. Rameriz and Beilock (2011) confirmed that the technique of emotional writing can be used to combat any stressful situation and was not limited to anxiety.

For more on this topic, you can watch this short PBS video[4] or search online for the work of Dr. Sian L. Beilock.

Additional strategies to combat negative emotions

There are myriad methods for counteracting negative emotions. The following introduces several strategies and resources where you can find supports that work best for your child.

Additional useful strategies to try with your child:

* Immediately start counting slowly from one to twenty and picture a smile in your head or view an actual picture of someone you know laughing or smiling a big smile.

* Write down your emotion or draw it.

* Walk away from the situation.

* Interrupt the emotion by turning on a really happy song and sing along or hum a happy tune.

* Do a series of 15 jumping jacks or squat thrusts—feel the positive adrenalin response.

---

4   www.pbs.org/wgbh/nova/body/sian-beilock.html

If your child is just beginning to recognize and deal with emotions, there are many really effective and free online resources to teach children about emotions.[5]

TECHNIQUES TO FOSTER EMPATHY

Having empathy for others is a critical skill for developing and sustaining social relationships. Empathy is not a condition a person has or does not have, but rather is a feeling or emotion that can be learned. There are many degrees of empathy and it can be taught to children if they are experiencing difficulty understanding others' feelings. This section describes strategies to teach empathy such as modeling empathic behavior and exercises in perspective taking.

Mindblindness

Within the condition of autism, a term has been created called mindblindness. This term was first postulated by Baron-Cohen (1985) as lack of theory of mind (ToM) as a way to explain the lack of obvious empathy or ability to embrace another person's perspective observed in many children with autism. However, I have seen children who have severe forms of autism express empathy by approaching someone who is crying and putting their arms around that person to console them. I have seen children apologize after causing a person pain because they recognized that they had hurt them. Some children may require more structured programs to strengthen their empathetic skills, and there are ways to do this.

---

5   I suggest the following: www.autismteachingstrategies.com; www.teacherspayteachers.com; www.do2learn.com; www.kimscounselingcorner.com; www.schoolsparks.com; www.teachertreasures.com; www.lighthouse-press.com; www.freeprintablebehaviorcharts.com; www.danielrechtschaffen.com

The first step in helping a child become empathic is to surround them with people who believe the child is capable of understanding and expressing empathy. When children experiences secure positive emotional attachments, they are more likely to demonstrate empathy and sympathy and offer help to others in distress (Kestenbaum, Farber, and Sroufe 1989). The following is an example of this method.

SUSAN

Susan often talks about her daughter's ability to express concern and caring for others, yet she has been told that her daughter lacks empathy as part of her diagnosis. On their way home from school, her daughter wanted to go to a familiar fast food restaurant and Susan said no. Susan was tired and wasn't feeling well. Immediately, her daughter began to tantrum, throwing her shoes and yelling. When Susan told her daughter she was feeling sick and she needed to rest, her daughter immediately stopped, became quiet, and then asked Susan if she needed a shoulder massage. Her daughter clearly understood that Susan was ill and was able to think of a strategy that might make her feel better. She was able to put herself in Susan's shoes, understand her mother's perspective, and express concern for her condition. In addition, she devised a solution to help her.

Perspective taking: putting yourself in someone else's shoes

Empathy is more than perspective taking or putting "yourself" in another's shoes. True empathy requires that you feel from the other person's perspective. Perspective taking was first illustrated by the classic Sally Anne false-belief test (Baron-Cohen, Leslie and Fitch 1985) in which a child predicts the behavior of a puppet that has seen an object hidden under one location, and then doesn't then see the object being moved to another location.

The child observing the puppet, if taking the perspective of the puppet, should predict that the puppet will look in the location that it first observed the object being hidden. The puppet would not know that the object was moved, because it did not see that action. If the child predicts that the puppet would somehow know the object was moved, and chooses the second location, they fail at perspective taking. Perspective taking, feeling like the other person would feel, is important for sharing, turn taking, and establishing and keeping friends; it's the hallmark of empathy. Strategies for teaching perspective taking are described in the next section.

Methods for teaching perspective taking

Perspective taking can be practiced by visually sequencing the main points of a story or sequencing of an observed situation leading up to why the person might be feeling a particular emotion such as sadness, fear, happiness, confusion, and so on. For example, if the child is watching a little league game and the last child up to bat strikes out, losing the game for the team, the child who swung the bat would most likely be feeling disappointed that they let their team down. This would be an opportunity for the child who has autism to say some kind words to that child such as, "I'm sorry you lost, you will get them next time." The child with autism needs to be able to put themself into the batter's shoes. What does it feel like to lose or let someone down? They must realize that this feeling is what is being experienced by the batter.

There are many opportunities during the course of the day for a child to learn about what another might be feeling, and what to say to another person that demonstrates they understand that person's feelings—empathy. This is how children learn to be socially in tune with each other. I would advise keeping an "emotions journal" that documents real experiences by emotion—sad/disappointed, happy, mad, frustrated, scared/anxious, and so on—and write down or use icons about what to say to a person who experiences these emotions. Review the journal on a regular basis, and practice being empathetic. Because children with autism don't always recognize facial expressions, you will need to practice recognizing and labeling these expressions.

Start building a library of everyday scenarios that you and your child can review together. These can be made up of real experiences that occur or stories or movies that you watch together. When real life situations occur, you can reference this library to highlight similarities and differences in the scenarios. Studies confirm that children perform better on perspective-taking tasks when families talk about these topics at home.

Another method for teaching perspective taking is modeling how to be empathetic through the use of video-modeling or videotaping a person demonstrating the desired behavior, and then dramatically highlighting the situation that demonstrates empathy. This is a good technique and can be regularly practiced in school or at home (LeBlanc and Coates 2003). Movies, role-playing, and social stories can be used to teach perspective taking by exploring what the character of the story might be feeling or thinking.

This section illustrated the importance of teaching empathy skills as a component of emotional understanding that leads to better self-regulation. It is critical for children with autism to not only be in better touch with their own emotions in order to regulate their behavior but to also be able to relate to what others are feeling and why. The final section of this chapter will explore self-efficacy and techniques to help build self-efficacy in children with autism.

TECHNIQUES TO FOSTER SELF-EFFICACY

Self-efficacy is the belief that you have in your skills to perform a task. It's not about how well you perform the task but more about the belief in your skills to accomplish the task. Some people, even if they perform very poorly time after time, may be highly self-efficacious and continually think they will do well regardless of past failures. This belief inspires them to continue to try in spite of initial defeat. The following section further defines the concept of self-efficacy and how it relates to the difficulties experienced by children with autism. Tips to boost self-efficacy are also offered.

Self-efficacy is an important consideration when emotional self-regulation is a goal because a child must first believe that can perform a task before they can begin to self-regulate. If they feel stressed immediately because they do not believe in their skills, then it will be difficult to self-regulate. Bandura (1986) defined self-efficacy as "people's judgment of their capabilities to organize and execute courses of action required to attain designated types of performances" (p.391). He noted that efficacious learners persist longer, tend not to avoid challenging tasks, and strive to become aware of what they need for a successful learning experience. Children's performance expectations influence their persistence, achievement, and aspirations (Bandura 1982). Children will likely become less efficacious and more anxious about learning after repeated negative experiences, such as poor or mismatched instruction, continued personal failure, and negative attitudes from adults and peers. Once a child has experienced many negative situations, their perceptions of their capabilities (self-efficacy) are negatively affected, leading to inferior images and abilities, which result in negative attitudes toward overall learning and poor performance (Czerniak and Chiarelott 1990). Conversely, experiences that contribute to a positive sense of self-efficacy lead to improved images of self and ability in positive attitudes toward learning and improved performance.

A child with a high degree of self-efficacy believes in their ability to organize their thoughts and the task at hand such that they believe that they can be successful. Self-efficacy is different than self-esteem in that self-esteem is related to a sense of self-worth, whereas self-efficacy is related to performance on tasks or activities. Self-efficacy has to do with a person's belief in their skills. Low self-efficacy in autism can come from high levels of anxiety, from feeling overwhelmed, or from continuous negative adult or peer feedback. The child's response to feelings of low self-efficacy can be seen as refusal to attempt a task, loss of motivation or giving up, anxiety when asked to do something, being afraid of making a mistake, or reduced effort overall. A child with low self-efficacy gives up earlier than those with high self-efficacy (Bandura 1993; Schunk and Zimmerman 2007).

Believing you can accomplish what you want to accomplish is one of the most important factors in succeeding. Helping a child with autism by using encouragement and positive support is particularly important as many of these children have experienced failure. Teaching the child to complete their work more independently, which requires learning how to sequence and organize, is a lifelong skill and also helps to build self-efficacy. Like the protagonist in *The Little Engine that Could*, a child who is equipped with an unwavering belief in their abilities and capacity to accomplish will continue to try until they accomplish what they set out to accomplish.

Bandura (1977) stated, "People see the extraordinary feats of others, but not the unwavering commitment and countless hours of perseverant effort that produced them" (p.119). Confidence, effort, and persistence are more powerful and a better predictors than ability (Dweck 2000). Some children with autism persist in areas that make them extraordinary in their knowledge or skills on a particular subject or activity. We need to help systematically broaden their skills and knowledge each day with support, kindness, and encouragement. We need our children to have a high degree of self-efficacy, as they will face many extraordinary challenges in their lives.

Tips for parents on fostering self-efficacy

Below are several do's and don'ts that can be helpful to parents and teachers when building a child's self-efficacy.

* Remember, the brain actually learns from failure and setbacks; the goal is ask yourself what you will do differently next time, and set out to do that. Do not try to avoid or protect your child from failure—help them embrace problems and not run away or shy away from them.

* Researchers at Columbia University suggest that you should praise your child's efforts versus praising their ability. If you tell your child that they are "very smart or very intelligent," it seems to induce fear of failure versus praising your child for their effort and encouraging them to try regardless of the outcome, which instills confidence.

* Always be sincere in your praise for efforts, and raise the bar as your child achieves more. Children know when we are sincere in our comments.

* When the child experiences failure, point how where their strengths were—be specific such as, "you really made excellent eye contact during the interview" or "your batting was excellent." Devise a plan to work on the weaker points for the next time.

* Teach through example—you need to demonstrate how you persevere even when you experience failure. Talk about these situations.

If you don't have the children's book, *The Little Engine that Could*, there is a YouTube video of the classic tale.[6] The first brief version of the tale was released in 1906, and appropriately titled, "Thinking One Can." I strongly suggest that as a parent or a person supporting a child with autism you watch this quick

---

6   www.youtube.com/watch?v=SiV0tj2lr00

half hour production by yourself. You also need a sense of self-efficacy, I CAN, as you raise and support your child. Keep this simple, yet extraordinary tale on hand for yourself and your child, or write your own version of the story adding new chapters as you succeed through your life's journey.

The Little Engine ends the story by tooting, "I did it, and it was worth it!"; that my friends, is how our stories should go.

EMOTIONAL REGULATION

1   4   7
_____

Little knowledge   *Very knowledgeable*

One strategy I would like to try:
_____

Chapter 7

ENERGY
REGULATION

Theresa Hamlin
with Nicole Kinney, DPT

This chapter is about rhythms and balance. Every human body thrives on naturally occurring rhythms. We all need to move and we all need to sleep so we can live, think, and learn. Now let's talk about regulating our energy to get the most out of our bodies and minds.

EXERCISE

We will start with exercise because so many children with autism that we see at The Center do not get enough exercise or movement during their daily routines. Contrary to popular belief and understanding, exercise is not just for weight control and making us more buff. In the next few paragraphs, you will see how important exercise is to your brain and your ability to function. Daily exercise is imperative for children with autism for many reasons, but most importantly because of its beneficial effect on stress reduction. Considering the positive effect of exercise on stress reduction, parents and teachers should be exercising right along with their child.

Exercise has a major effect on the brain, on inflammation, and especially on what we are broadly calling stress, or better, toxic stress. Ratey (2008), a psychiatrist and professor at Harvard Medical School and a researcher at The Center For Discovery, wrote a book called *Spark*, which details the effects of exercise on the brain and traces this back to our hunter-gatherer days when people moved 8 to 14 miles a day on average. Yes, humans actually moved all day long, mainly for survival, but nonetheless this demonstrates that we have built-in equipment in the form of our body structure to move each day for extended periods of time. This is important to children with autism for the following reasons.

In his book, Ratey talks about the multiple effects that exercise has on our neurochemicals, the chemicals that keep our bodies and brains functioning and alert (Ratey and Manning 2014). These chemicals help to keep our brains, emotions, and ability to learn and perform at an optimal level. For children with autism, exercise helps to decrease aggression, self-abuse, distractibility, anxiety, mood instability, and attention difficulties. These are the problems that parents worry about the most because they seem to be the ones that interfere with the child's daily routines and ability to learn in school. Currently, Ratey and The Center for Discovery staff are studying the benefits of exercise for children with the most significant needs, a group frequently overlooked in scientific literature.

We know that exercise acts by changing the neurochemicals, the neurotransmitters like norpeinephrine, serotonin, dopamine, gamma-aminobatric acid (GABA), and glutamate. Exercise also improves the concentration of another important group of chemicals called neuro growth factors, which are very important in managing our brains immediately. Exercise helps our brains to grow. All of these benefits help us be ready and able to learn!

We have learned much of this during the last 20 years of scientific studies that look at how exercise impacts our brains. We have accumulated evidence that exercise is as good as antidepressants in helping mood—both elevating it and stabilizing it. We also know that exercise is an important way to keep our attention fixed and focused, which has been illustrated by its use in helping to control impulsive behavior.

We now have an abundance of evidence that exercise optimizes our ability to learn, remember, and use information productively. A 2011 review by the Mayo Clinic (Ahlskog *et al.* 2011) demonstrated that of more than 1600 scientific papers on the effect of exercise and cognition there was a profound positive effect of exercise on keeping our brains growing rather than eroding with age, making us smarter, and allowing us to use our brains most effectively.

Similarly, Ratey (Ratey and Manning 2014) contended that exercise has an effect on learning in three complementary ways. First, it makes for a better learner. Children and adults who exercise are more attentive, less fidgety, more motivated, less impulsive, and better able to overcome stress. So that makes for a better learner. In addition, exercise causes our 100 billion brain cells to be better nourished by the wide variety of neurotransmitters, growth factors, and hormones that encourage our brain cells to grow and thus wire in memories more easily. Finally, exercise is the most effective human activity that we know of that has a positive effect on growing new brain cells. All these influences make it easier for any of us, and especially the child with autism, to learn new behaviors and extinguish unhelpful and disruptive behaviors.

Exercise for children with maladaptive behaviors

Research has indicated that a systematic physical exercise program practiced before learning by children with maladaptive and aggressive behaviors can result in increased attention, appropriate responding, and time on task, along with a decrease in inappropriate behaviors (Kern, Koegel, and Dunlap 1984; Watters and Watters 1980). More vigorous bouts of physical activity have led to positive behavior changes when compared to less vigorous or light physical activity (Lang *et al.* 2010a). Conversely, when children with aggressive behaviors weren't able to be active, their behaviors became exacerbated (McGimsey and Favell 1988). This is important to understand, as I have seen many children with autism who have aggressive behaviors sitting in cubicles in classrooms with little opportunity for exercise. Children are also often punished for bad behavior and made to sit. If you want to correct the bad behavior, sitting is not the answer. You are better off having the child start to run or do a fast set of jumping jacks or other vigorous activity when you see them getting upset. This can actually stop or dampen the initiation of the full-blown stress response and subsequent negative behavior.

Vigorous exercise for the treatment and reduction of maladaptive behavior is defined as 20-minutes or longer aerobic workout five times a week. Mild exercise, like walking at a slow or normal pace, seems to have little effect on behavior change for children with autism (Oriel *et al.* 2011).

When we think about weight gain, we know that many children with autism experience this and are overweight or obese because of a sedentary lifestyle, a poor diet, and sometimes because of side effects from medication. Statistics have suggested that children with autism are an alarming 40 percent more likely to be overweight and obese when compared to their peers without autism. This should be cause for concern, as this extra weight takes a toll on the body and the brain and adds extra stress to the system (Curtin *et al.* 2010).

It's important that children with autism be allowed the opportunity to participate in vigorous exercise routines during the day because it is the single most important activity that demands the most nerve cells to be used in the brain at one time. Think of the brain as an organ that needs to get into shape to function successfully. I like to call it "thinking shape." Zumba, dance routines, and "follow the leader" types of vigorous exercise are among the best because they demand that nerve cells fire.

According to Ratey and Manning (2014), when nerve cells fire, you create more neurotransmitters. The result is like taking Prozac and Ritalin, because you increase the concentration of norepinephrine, dopamine and serotonin in the brain. The results of exercising are better focus, better control, and less impulsivity. For the first time, the American Psychiatric Association has included exercise as a treatment for depression. It is not just the population-based evidence advantages; we have solid data about the biochemical changes in blood-tests and how our genes change as a result of exercise. The Institute of Medicine has also recommended that exercise occur in schools every day and should be considered a core component of the curriculum. The national guidelines for physical activity for people of all age groups suggest a minimum of 60 minutes a day of moderate to vigorous physical activity (United States Department of Health and Human Services 2010).

There has been an explosion of research over the past few years confirming that exercise boosts brainpower, especially in the areas of attention, organization, and planning, reduces depression, and enhances the immune response. Bassuk, Church and Manson (2013) are now detailing the positive changes that occur with exercise at the level of the cells and molecules for specific conditions like atherosclerosis and diabetes.

The science of exercise

When a muscle is active during exercise, the body responds by excreting a chemical called IGR-I, which travels through the blood stream to the brain. This chemical increases the production of another really important chemical called brain-derived neurotropic factor (BDNF), which Ratey (2008) called "miracle grow for the brain." With this chemical, the brain's nerve cells branch out, join together, and communicate in new ways. Just and colleagues (Just *et al.* 2007) noted that children with autism have under-connectivity in the brain, especially in the frontal lobe. Kramer and Erickson (2007) demonstrated that exercise causes the frontal lobes—the center for higher order thinking and self-regulation—to increase in size by creating new neuronal connections.

Fernando Gomez-Pinilla (2011) documented that exercise, in combination with select diets that contain Omega 3s, plant-based food, and saturated fats, enhanced the production of BDNF in the brain. In another study, Albeck and colleagues (Albeck *et al.* 2006) demonstrated that rats that were forced to exercise, versus those that exercised voluntarily, showed an even greater benefit of BDNF. In other words, exercising while stressed had a very positive effect as did eating select foods and exercising to increase BDNF.

According to Ratey and Manning (2014), the newest and most exciting research on exercise is currently being conducted using lab rats. Researchers are discovering that when a person exercises, they build up nerves cells that both excite and control the level of arousal and alertness. Not only is a person able to get more aroused and excited, but at the same time they have better control. There are two different sets of nerve cells being created at the same time. This is the reason why people who exercise are better able to control stress and anxiety and experience fewer anxiety attacks. They build nerve cells as well.

For whatever reason, when people hear the word exercise, many think hard work and that it is not for them. Even schools downplay the need for and benefits of exercise, yet these same institutions complain that children are not paying attention and that they are too wriggly and distracted in class. The problem is that we need exercise in order to pay attention, but it seems that for most exercise needs to be fun and easy so it can be incorporated into a child's day.

The ENERGym and exercise breaks

My colleagues and I have designed a simple and fun program—ENERGym—to promote health and enhance aerobic functioning, balance, core strength, coordination, and overall body strength for children with autism. It is completed in a circuit design, where children experience short, vigorous bouts of exercise as they move from one activity to the next. Given the predictable routine of a circuit, the children who have autism find the routine organizing and calming. They can independently complete the program once they understand what is expected at each station. And best of all, they ask for ENERGym time.

Picture cards or short videos of someone using the equipment or completing the exercise routine in the ENERGym can help remind the child of the expected behavior at each station. Each station should have a timer that can be set to keep track of time spent at each station. Time can increase as the child's strength and endurance increase. Begin with two minutes per station and the expectation that the child will eventually spend five minutes working at each station.

Although many children with autism may be very active, they often lack coordination and core strength, the ability to maintain their balance when it is challenged, and the ability to motor plan, which is the ability to take in sensory information in order to successfully plan and then carry out a new motor skill. These issues make it difficult for children with autism to excel in many gross and fine motor tasks requiring coordination. According to a recent study by Piochon *et al.* (2014), the cerebellum—the motor and coordination center of the brain—is not functioning well in many children with autism. Exercises, such as those promoted through the ENERGym, Burpee, or Bosu break, will strengthen the cerebellum and other key large muscles in the body.

Burpee

What's a burpee, you ask? A burpee is a squat thrust that ends in a jump and it is a really easy way to incorporate vigorous exercise into your day. I recommend that classroom teachers give their children a burpee break after each period and before all academic lessons. Parents can also call for burpee breaks throughout the day, especially before any activity that might be stressful. It's designed to get the mind and body energized, and it also promotes calmness and attention. You can find out how to do a burpee in "The ABCs of ENERGym" later in this book.

BOSU ball

A BOSU ball is basically a therapy or stability ball that has been cut in half and attached to a rigid base. It is a great balance-training tool. BOSU stands for "both sides up" because you can perform balance exercises on the half-ball side or turn the piece of equipment over and perform exercises on the rigid base. These can easily be stored in the classroom and readily taken out for movement breaks.

What is a BOSU break? There are many exercises that can be performed on the BOSU to promote balance (see "The ABCs of ENERGym" later in this book). I recommend using the half-ball side for these breaks. Here are a couple of suggested exercises that can easily be done during a short movement break:

1. marching in place while standing on the BOSU

2. squats—have the child stand on the BOSU and ask them to bend their knees as if they were going to sit back in a chair. Keeping their arms extended in front of them will help them maintain their balance as they are beginning this type of exercise.

ENERGym

ENERGym is an easy program to set up in the home or school environment. We all benefit from exercise, making it a terrific activity for the entire family and classroom.

To create an ENERGym, your home or classroom will need the following:

* a BOSU ball for balance and core strengthening

* a bounce disc, used as an alternative to a trampoline. The bounce disc gives added stability and in turn greater sensory input because its base is made of wood with six vinyl covered durable springs underneath the top surface. If a bounce disc is not available a mini trampoline may be a substitute

* two or three mats for exercises like burpees, crunches, hip thrusts, modified, or non-modified push-ups

* a balance beam or tape line on the floor if a balance beam is not available

* an aerobic step or two that can be placed on top of each other or the bottom step of a staircase if an aerobic step is not readily available

* soft weights of 1–5 lbs made from rubber

* a 30–36 inch ball that can be used for sitting at the kitchen table as well for exercise.

Set up six to eight separate exercise activities in a circular layout. I have found that when children are first introduced to ENERGym, visual markers on the floor are helpful to direct children from one station to the next. An arrow made out of tape is an easy visual. Eventually, the child can be taught to rotate around the circle without visual cues, completing each activity before moving to the next. A timer or count down strip for the number of repetitions may be used to indicate to the child how much exercise is required per station before moving to the next.

There are many options for the actual exercises to use at each station; a mix of activities that promote aerobic fitness, balance, core strengthening, coordination, and generalized strengthening is best. These are the ABCs of ENERGym, which include aerobic, balance, core, coordination, and strengthening exercises, and can be found later in the book.

Walking

Sometimes we forget that simply walking has tremendous health benefits that go beyond basic health. Consciously walking, whether fast or slow, de-stresses the brain and body. It's as good as meditation. Conscious walking takes practice because you need to stay present and focused on your steps. Try walking with a focus on your footsteps from your car, train, or whatever transport you may use to get from home to work and back again. Lift one foot and bend at the knee; bring the whole leg forward and step down onto the ground heel first; repeat with the other foot.

Practice this as slowly as you can in the beginning. Avoid the temptation to use your phone or other multimedia. In the beginning, give yourself a little extra time to arrive at your destination. Be conscious and take note of how you feel once you arrive at your destination. You should begin to feel a sense of calmness, unless you didn't give yourself enough time and you're late for work. Repeat this for at least ten days, and you will begin to feel the benefits of this simple action of walking with intention. Once you have mastered conscious walking, you can pick up the pace.

SLEEP

Similar to exercise, sleep is now understood to be essential for brain and body health. Conversely, losing sleep or not getting enough sleep can be detrimental to long- and short-term health.

This shouldn't come as a surprise, as sleep affects our ability to cope with stress, stay calm, keep focused, learn new information, and fight off infection. If you think about it, sleep deprivation has been used as a form of torture in war, causing prisoners to lose their sense of reality.

Clinically, the first thing that a doctor will ask about when suspecting a psychiatric condition like depression or bi-polar disorder is your sleep pattern. Sleeping too little, too much, or experiencing interrupted sleep is detrimental to your overall mental and physical health. In people who lack sleep, there is a clear indication of stress, as the cortisol and blood glucose levels are elevated indicative of a body under stress. These levels will return to normal once the individual's sleep pattern is restored to a healthy level.

Sleep and food

Sleep also affects our metabolism and how our food gets digested. Recently, it was discovered that part of the problem for people who are have trouble losing weight, is that they don't sleep well. Lack of sleep is a culprit in hypertension, obesity, and cardiovascular disease (Greer, Goldstein and Walker 2013; Kondracki 2012). The best advice for improved sleeping relative to food is to follow a well-balanced, plant-based diet that is also rich in protein, moderate in carbohydrates, and low in fat. This kind of diet was promoted in Chapter 5 of this book. A healthy diet should ensure an adequate supply of micronutrients and generally improve mood and energy throughout the day (Benson and Donohoe 1999).

Sleep and the brain

Tononi and Cirelli (2014) suggested that during sleep neuronal connections made during the day are actually weakened and not strengthened, as previously believed. The brain is actually making room in its "inbox" for the next day by eliminating waste. The goal of sleep is to prevent the brain from becoming overwhelmed with all the new information experienced during the day. Sleep is essential, as it restores the brain to a receptive baseline state so it is possible to function with a clear and open mind the next day. Sleep is also necessary for the brain if it is to remodel itself in response to its experiences. The body revolves around balanced sleep and wake cycles. Children with autism oftentimes have trouble with that balance, since both the quality and quantity of their sleep can be decreased.

Sleep and children with autism

A study conducted by Humpreys and colleagues (Humpreys *et al.* 2014) revealed that children with autism slept less than their typically developing peers. They had more frequent interrupted sleep, waking up more often during the night then their peers. Likewise, a study by the UC Davis Mind Institute found that children with autism wake up in the middle of the night significantly more frequently than their typically developing peers regardless of the severity of autism (Krakowiak *et al.* 2008). Malow and McGrew (2008) noted that when sleep is not a problem, children with autism demonstrated fewer emotional problems and better social interactions. We have found that about 75 percent of the children admitted into our programs experience notable sleep problems. According to Krakowiak and colleagues (2008), 40 to 80 percent of children with autism experience sleep disturbance. One of the major concerns for families is that when their child doesn't sleep, they don't sleep either. Entire families can suffer from sleep deprivation when one child doesn't sleep. This can take its toll by affecting everyone's health and well-being. Regulating sleep is essential to transform how well a person with autism performs during the day and to positively affect health.

Here is the number of hours sleep experts recommend for everyone at different ages to lead healthy lives:

Infants ages 3–11 months	14–15 hours
Toddlers ages 1–3 years	12–14 hours
Preschoolers ages 3–5 years	11–13 hours
School-aged ages 5–10 years	10–11 hours
Teens	9–10 hours

What you can do to establish a healthy sleep routine

Children with autism exert a tremendous amount of energy all day long as they attend to everything in their environments. They have difficulty processing social and complex information, which can be exhausting. Developing a bedtime routine is essential to help a child regulate sleep.

A bedtime routine, beginning about one hour prior to sleeping, should be one that is consistent and relaxing without the addition of new information or stressful activities. Foods and even drinks, especially sugary or caffeinated ones, should be avoided right before bed as they can result in interrupted sleep. Sleep should occur at the same time each night. It is healthy for the body to have routine and consistency, including weekends and holidays. The body doesn't discriminate between days of the week.

Quiet activities, such as reading and listening to soft music or stories that are not too dramatic, are good activities for pre-bedtime. Activities to avoid are those with too much stimulation. The brain and body should be calmed down during this phase of the day. Once in bed, the room temperature should be on the cooler side but comfortable. The room should be dark without the intrusion of clock lights or computer screens, including hand-held computer games. Falling asleep with the TV on is not advisable.

This routine should be exercised nightly. Sleep time should be treated as sacred. I can't emphasize enough how critical sleep is to learning and daily functioning. As we try to cram more and more into our days, we have become a society that devalues the importance of sleep. It's not healthy for anyone, but it can be detrimental for a child with autism.

DAILY RHYTHMS

If you take only one lesson from this book, remember that keeping the same basic rhythmic schedule of when you eat, wake up, go to sleep, exercise, and eliminate body waste is one of the most important things you can do with and for your child. You are helping them regulate their way to success. During the day, unexpected things will always happen, but the daily anchor events should remain as constant as possible. Children with autism need predictability and routine in their schedules; these elements are essential for a healthier body and mind.

Rhythm of time

There is another type of ubiquitous rhythm: the rhythm of time. The rhythmic beats of our daily life are important considerations when helping a child calm their body and mind. For all of us, the beat of our world seems to be getting faster, with little time to accomplish all we wish we could on a daily basis. Rechtschaffen (1996), M.D. and author of *Time Shifting*, spoke about a change being experienced by all of us living in modern society, where life's rhythms and time seem to be accelerated; as a result, stress has started to become more pervasive. According to Rechtschaffen, even prisoners who are incarcerated for life feel that they don't have enough time to accomplish what they need to do in a day.

Many of us in society live on the verge of fight or flight, the body's autonomic nervous system's response to stress. Road rage is a relatively new phenomenon; it only takes a minor incident to tip us over the stress point so we become completely enraged at a fellow driver.

About a week ago, I was in the audience for a series of musical dance performances by a fairly large group of students who had autism. The ten performances were set to a fast-paced, hip-hop beat. The performers had practiced for weeks and were excited and a bit nervous to finally perform for a large audience of peers and family. The younger children aged 5–8 performed the first two sets, which were quite enjoyable as the beat of the music was set to the slow motion of the Itsy Bitsy Spider. Then it was time for the teenagers to perform. It was quite a feat for teenagers with complex and severe forms of autism to come up on the stage and perform in sync with their peers and in front of their parents and classmates. They were clearly excited yet comfortable on stage. The beat of the music picked up considerably, as did the audience participation with enthusiastic clapping, when they performed the song "Happy" by Pharrell Willams. As the volume of noise and audience participation increased, the stereotypical rocking and jumping behaviors, rarely seen any more in the children with autism who were in the audience, began to be pervasive.

In a matter of three songs, many of the audience participants were overly excited, rocking, and jumping, and some of them were beginning to run. They had reached their tipping points of overexcitement and dysregulation. They were in full fight or flight mode. The teens who were performing were unaffected by the rhythm. They performed with control and composure and were beautifully in sync with each other. In the audience, however, the teachers were taking children out of the theater into quieter spaces, trying to get them to calm down and also allowing themselves to calm down. After the concert, the staff held a meeting to discuss what they had experienced and put strategies in place for upcoming performances that would ensure the children would not become overly aroused by them. It was a good teachable moment for everyone involved.

Dr. Rechtschaffen spoke about the above-mentioned phenomenon in his book (1996). The rhythm or the beat of the external world quickly becomes entrained in us. The faster the pace we set or we experience, the faster our body responds. Try counting your heartbeat or breathing while stuck in traffic or when listening to rock music. Your heart and breathing rate will increase above the normal 60–70 beats per minute. It is easy to get swept up in a hectic pace and to become exhausted and short tempered. Even worse, those around you can become entrained with you.

We see this phenomenon in children when using heart rate monitors. Once one child or staff becomes stressed, the others are soon to follow unless there is a conscious calming intervention. Our bodies are not built to work at a continuous fast and stressful pace, which can be seen in unhealthy long-term outcomes. Outcomes are poorer for those who experience constant stress and don't allow their brains and bodies to relax.

As a person supporting a child with autism, you need to take the time to relax and experience surroundings that are calmer and require less emotional energy. I understand that this isn't always possible. The good news is that it doesn't need to be. A little bit of calmness through consistency goes a long way.

As discussed in Chapter 6, I would highly encourage you to practice mindfulness during the day. Take time for yourself by practicing deep breathing for three minutes, three to five times per day or walk slowly and intentionally when going from your car to work, or find a quiet place that is a retreat—a place that has an external rhythm that is slow. Try relaxing listening to soft 60-beats per minute music while you cook or clean. I listen to Reggae music, much of which is pulsed at 60 beats per minute. Bob Marley's "Survival" album is my favorite. But of course if

Reggae isn't your favorite, there are many more options with 60-beat music. You can just search online to discover your options.

In a study by Gomez and Danuser (2007), it was discovered that music with a fast, accentuated, staccato beat induced faster breathing and heart rate than did slower beats. I would carefully consider the music you choose for what it is you are trying to accomplish. It really makes a difference—remember your body entrains to your surroundings and others entrain to you. It has been demonstrated that many children with autism have higher rhythmic resting states, and can be anxious much of the time. You will benefit yourself and your child if you find a way to have a counter calming rhythm.

SUMMARY

Energy regulation is about balance and rhythm in our life using the external environments or conscious strategies to regulate our bodies and our brains. I would recommend that you begin to take notice of your rhythms and your child's rhythms— become conscious of the beat of your life. If it's too fast, slow it down. Find ways to entrain to a 60–70 beat per minute daily relaxation activity.

ENERGY REGULATION

1	4	7
Little knowledge		Very knowledgeable

One strategy I would like to try:

_____

PART 3

Chapter 8

HOW DO I KNOW IF THE ESSENTIALS ARE WORKING?

What to Keep Track of

In this chapter I will share with you the critical components to track daily that will help guide interventions and provide insights into what's working and what's not working for your child. What you have learned from this book is that there are critical factors that affect children with autism and that these can be regulated.

Getting back to Grandpa Norbert, as Chief Engineer, he knowingly set the controls on the critical parts of the tug's engine. The tug couldn't function without his knowledge about the tug's engine and about the ever-changing environmental conditions facing the tug. Once he optimized everything for the daily conditions, the regulators automatically managed the engine and its stressors. Life is about actively regulating stressors—the parts of the day that challenge us. For children with autism, there are many parts of the day that can cause undue stress. Our bodies constantly strive to be in harmony or allostatis as it's called in science. It's important to help a child with autism regulate their days so that their bodies and minds can achieve harmony.

In order to do his job, my grandfather had to monitor and collect data to ensure things were working properly and in harmony. What I have suggested to you is this book is that you can do the same for yourself and your child. You can identify the critical factors to monitor and adjust to ensure optimal functioning. Let's explore what those factors are and how to keep track of them.

There are key indicators to look for in your child that can tell you about how well they are functioning. These are things that you want to keep track of as they can indicate signs of trouble in the body and brain.

In this chapter, you will learn the best methods for collecting data, what data is best to collect, and how to think about the data once it has been collected.

COLLECTING INFORMATION

Parents and educators struggle trying to keep track of everything that needs to be done for the child who has autism. However, information about how the child is functioning is very helpful and necessary to collect and share with all those who are trying to help. As you read in Chapter 3, there are many people intimately involved in the care, support, and education of a child who has autism. The information about how your child is feeling and performing on a daily basis helps guide the team toward developing the best interventions for the best outcomes for everyone involved.

There are a few strategies and techniques that I recommend for keeping track of essential information including creating a calendar, journaling, and using data tracking devices. These are strategies and techniques that can be naturally incorporated into the day. First, I recommend beginning with writing daily notes in a journal.

Before you say, I don't have time to write, let me explain. I'm not suggesting that you write a novel, or even complete sentences. On the contrary, I recommend keeping it simple. Your time is limited, and you want to see just the essentials.

Journaling

A journal can be calendar based and have a simple design to keep track of daily information that you will refer back to. Read on to learn how to keep this simple.

You can begin with documenting on a number scale how your day was and how your child's day was—nothing elaborate. This can be easily expressed by a number from 1–7; 1 being not good at all and 7 being excellent or couldn't have been better. To start this process you need to write a brief sentence describing what your worst day might look and feel like.

Conversely, do the same for what your best day might look and feel like. For example, one of the parents I work with told me that her worst day is when her daughter doesn't sleep, and as a result, she doesn't sleep. The day will then typically progress with a meltdown that lasts the entire morning. She becomes frazzled, exhausted, and angry, and so does her daughter. The opposite end, a 7, is when she and her daughter get a good night's sleep, waking up is easy, and getting off to school is a breeze. The rest of the day is typically uneventful and even fun.

Don't be discouraged if you rarely have days that are 7s right now. Most parents don't; it's one of the main reasons I decided to write this book. These two extremes—1 and 7—are now your guideposts by which to judge each day. By entering a number reflective of your day you will quickly get a sense of how many really good days and how many not so good days you are having. Entering one number a day assumes your day is affected by how your child is doing. You can enter two separate numbers if you like—one for your child's day and one for your day. Either approach is fine.

Armed with a month or two of information, you can then begin to figure out which days are good and which days are not so good. Over time, you will begin to discover patterns. This information is very helpful, as you and your child will change over time. Some days, months, and years will be better than others.

When things are not so good, there may be ways to improve, which can emerge out of the data. This is just the beginning of gathering basic information that can really help you objectively help your child and yourself.

The calendar

Before thinking about what to keep track of, let's talk about the best system to use. I recommend continuing with a calendar-based, tracking system. I would buy or make a daily calendar that shows the entire month at a glance. Choose a calendar that is big enough to write on. There are several critical factors that you want to keep track of in a calendar, so the size of the calendar matters. My daily calendar has a day-by-day space that is big enough to write in.

Using a paper-based calendar may seem a little old fashioned, but not everyone has access to an electronic calendar on a platform that is big enough to view all factors in a month-by-month layout. Once you decide on a calendar, you can begin to gather information.

As noted already, the first piece of data you will enter on the calendar is a number from 1 to 7 to represent how your day went. This number should be added to the upper right corner of the particular day. If you chose to keep a number to represent your day and another number to represent your child's day, make sure to be consistent about where you write these numbers on the calendar. You may want to take the upper right corner to write your number representing your day, and your child's may be represented in the upper left opposite corner.

Data-recording devices

There are many data-recording technologies available from simple step counters to more elaborate, web-based, integrated tracking systems. These technologies are constantly emerging and appear to be getting more accurate. For home use, however, I recommend keeping it simple and inexpensive.

DAILY FUNCTIONS TO KEEP TRACK OF

In addition to the general information about your day and your child's day, I highly recommend keeping track of several other functions that occur on a routine basis. The following sections introduce some indicators that show how our bodies and brains are functioning.

Bowel elimination

A bowel movement log is one of the first elements I advise tracking because there is a high rate of GI problems in children with autism that often correlate with behavior problems. Bowel elimination problems are very common and linked to behavioral problems in children with autism. Keeping track of these patterns is a critical factor when trying to understand why your child may be exhibiting maladaptive behaviors as discussed in Chapter 5.

A simple big bold **B**, medium **B**, or little **b**, can be a useful way to track this. You can also write a b with a slash (b̸) to represent no bowel movement. Multiple bowel movements, such as 3**B** can be used to represent three large bowel movements during a day. If the bowel movement is unusual—diarrhea, foul smelling, or very hard and pellet-like stool—you can create and find simple graphics to note them. The Bristol Stool Chart, as shown on p.226, is very useful and is typically used by professionals in the medical field to describe bowel movements. Most important is that you keep track of your child's bowel pattern. You can then share this information with your child's doctor if there is a problem.

Sleep

Sleep is a vital function in overall health and well-being. It can affect a child's behavior, ability to attend, and ability to retain new information. Hours of sleep per night in particular are very important to track. We examined the reasons for this in Chapter 7.

Quality and quantity of sleep are both problems for children with autism; however, the most common type of sleep disorder in these children is insomnia. In order to track sleep, I usually draw a cloud on the calendar with a number representing the number of hours slept that night. It's typically best to review a few weeks or a month of sleep to begin to see if positive or negative patterns of sleep are occurring.

There are a number of devices using actigraphy and polysomnograpy that track sleep. If you Google "sleep tracking devices" you will find a number of current easy to use, wearable and non-wearable devices. It should be noted that not all devices are completely accurate, so you may need to test for accuracy by wearing the device yourself or speaking to a company representative.

If your child experiences a pattern of disrupted sleep or can't fall asleep, you should share this with your child's doctor. Although quite common in autism, lack of sleep should be treated by discovering the root cause of the problem. Getting more vigorous exercise during the day and eating a wholefoods plant-based diet can make a difference in a better night's sleep. There are times when a physician may recommend a medication to support sleep.

I highly encourage you to track your own sleep patterns in this cloud. If you're not sleeping it will be very difficult to help your child. Your sleep matters as much as theirs.

Exercise

The amount of exercise your child gets during the day is also important to document. Children need to move to stay healthy and to learn. As discussed in Chapter 7, exercise supports learning and health and helps to decrease anxiety and the effects of stress.

Exercise can be represented by a number of minutes exercised a day. For example, 60E might be used to mean your child had 60 minutes of exercise that day. Keeping track of movement is a reminder that kids need to move to maintain their body and brain health. If your child moves a lot, this may not be necessary to track, but if they are sedentary or sitting much of their day, this should be tracked.

Children often sit for extended periods in school, so asking the teacher to report on movement is important. It is advisable that children get at least one hour a day of vigorous exercise in order to stay healthy. The more your child exercises the better, especially if they have a high level of stress.

Behavior

Behavior tracking is also really important. This can be very elaborate as dictated by behavioral support plans; for parents, however, a simpler tracking system is often the best. This may be represented by another scale of 1–7 for perceived severity of the behavior during the day. Alternatively, it may be a behavioral count. It is best to speak with professional staff to determine what is most appropriate for you and your child. The important thing is that knowing about the frequency and intensity of behaviors will aid in determining treatment techniques, especially for biomedical treatments. We sometimes equip families with portable cameras to capture behaviors on video. The video is then used to determine which behaviors are most important to track.

Food intake

Quality and quantity of food are important information to document, as they are the fuel source for the body and brain. This documentation doesn't need to be elaborate, nor does it need to fit on the calendar. I suggest a simple food log. You can randomly sample your child's eating patterns with this. By collecting data intermittently several times a month over several months, you will get a sense of your child's dietary habits. If you know everything your child eats and drinks on a daily basis, sampling may not be necessary. With this method, you should include any and all snacks or food rewards. Every bit of food counts. What we eat and drink affects functioning and health, so keeping a log is an important factor in determining an intervention strategy.

Time outdoors

Believe it or not, children are spending less time outdoors than they used to. The decline of children's outdoor play is often blamed on the advancement and availability of technology including television, computers, apps, and smartphones. While these changes have played a significant role in the decline of time outdoors, Clements (2004) noted that 85 percent of mothers she interviewed cited television viewing and 81 percent cited computer play as the culprit in not going outdoors. However, in the same survey, most of the mothers admitted that they themselves had restricted their children's outdoor play, mainly because of safety concerns, including fear of crime.

Safety is a major concern, and children will need to be supervised closely in the outdoor environment. For children with autism who wander, parks with perimeter fences are best. In more rural settings, boundaries should be clearly established and children will need to be closely monitored. The benefits, however, of being in the outdoors are well documented and well worth the effort.

Seizure activity (epilepsy)

Seizures in autism are quite common and were first documented by Leo Kanner in 1943. According to Shafali Jeste (2011) who conducted an extensive review of the literature, up to one third of children with autism also have co-occurring epilepsy. If your child has a seizure disorder, then it is important to keep track of when seizures occur, how long they last, and what type of seizure they are experiencing each time. Types and treatments of seizures are beyond the scope of this book; however, it is imperative that you keep track of seizures and speak with your child's neurologist if you suspect your child might have a seizure disorder.

Medications

I have not written extensively about medication in this book; however, I recognize that medication may be needed for medical and psychiatric conditions. The framework presented in this book is fundamental for establishing basic health; however, it will not totally eliminate the primary educational problems of children with autism. If the child has other underlying medical conditions such as a seizure disorder, psychiatric condition, or GI problems, they need to be treated. You and your child's doctors should work together to determine if they require medication to treat a medical issue. If medication is a part of your routine, I recommend that you keep track of the patterns in a medical log.

Medical information management

As noted throughout this book, children with autism have many co-occurring medical conditions that are managed by many different medical specialists. It is often left to the parent to organize, coordinate, and keep track of their child's appointments and results of tests and treatments. There can be literally volumes of information that parents carry with them from appointment to appointment. I recently met with a parent who came into my office carrying a huge shopping bag with three binders of reports about her child that she had beautifully organized into categories of problems. She said her major problem was carrying the binders as they were getting so heavy that she was thinking of getting a backpack so she could free up her hands to hold onto her son when he was with her. I suggest to parents who are struggling to keep their child's medical information together that there is a much better way to do this, which is not only beneficial as an organizational strategy, but also can be very helpful to your child's physicians as medical information is immediately available and prioritized for them.

Scores of electronic medical record (EMR) platforms are currently in use throughout the country. While clearly providing some very distinct advantages over traditional paper-based records, the major limitations of EMRs are complexity and a lack of portability. EMRs contain voluminous data collected at a single health care institution. Unfortunately, it is not possible to share the information among providers as a patient moves between various institutions for highly specialized care. This inability to share information about previous testing and medical treatments often leads to painful, expensive, and redundant testing. Inadequate historical information can also lead to treatment errors such as dangerous drug interactions.

During the past five years, we have used one of the commercially available EMRs to manage our on-site health information. However, many of our residents require specialized care on an intermittent basis and must be transferred to tertiary care centers. We have addressed the limitations of share-ability and portability by extracting essential medical data from our on-site EMR, combined it with medical information collected from off-site providers, and organized it into an intuitive, electronic health record containing important information from all providers that have cared for our residents. The record-sharing platform that we have chosen is also commercially available. The web-based, encrypted, organized information is immediately available to authorized individuals. Parents, and providers at institutions to which we transfer our residents, have found the program to be very beneficial for sharing complex and voluminous data from numerous medical providers.

PATTERNS EMERGE

Over time, patterns from the collective data will emerge. You may find that when your child did not sleep well, they exhibited more behaviors during the day. You may find that your child didn't sleep well when they were constipated. Each child and each situation is unique, and it is only by collecting information that you can determine what is and what is not working.

It should come as no surprise that your level of stress can easily influence your child's behavior. If you're upset, nervous, or anticipating a problem, a problem will almost certainly occur. Co-regulation is a major factor in working with children who have autism. It's really important to understand your own stressors, and make sure that you are taking measures to keep yourself calm.

Keep track of your own regulatory behaviors. For example, I wear a bracelet with wooden beads, Mala beads, that I call my calming bracelet. I use it to remind me to breathe deeply during the day, but it also serves to remind me that I have to take care of my health in general. As I practice my breathing, I begin to think about the amount of exercise I engaged in, what I ate and drank during the day, and so on. One simple bracelet leads to a daily cascade of thoughts intended to keep me conscious about my health.

SUMMARY

Collecting information provides you with objective information about how your child is functioning and feeling on a day-to-day basis and over time. The information should be used to guide decisions about what is working and what needs to change. It can also be highly informative to physicians who may be caring for the child. Physicians' time is limited and our children are complex, therefore an organized approach to the collection of information over time, presented in a consistent format, can really help physicians, clinicians, and educators better treat your child. Find a simple way to gather important information that suits your style. Usually, the easier it is to collect the more you will collect it—so keep it simple and be consistent.

Chapter 9

WHERE TO
BEGIN

This book has been written so that the ideas and strategies can be taught to a wide audience of parents and professionals. The underlying message is that children with autism are under tremendous and continuous pressure in the learning and social environments, and that pressure can cause undue stress on their bodies and brains, making learning and daily functioning difficult at best. You now have the knowledge and some suggested strategies to begin to reduce the burden of stress on your child and increase their health and vitality by regulating their experiences and environments. There is not one, single cure-all. The benefits of incorporating all the elements included in this book into daily life can be widely effective on the body, brain, and health and happiness. The greatest advantages of the strategies in this book is that most are free, they can be started immediately in your home, and they can benefit the whole family.

Teaching and talking to others about what you have learned is a powerful way to ensure your own learning. It helps solidify knowledge by committing it to long-term memory. In order to teach others though, you first need to reflect on and organize your own thoughts about the information in this book. I would encourage you to start the process of organization by thinking in chunks—that is, small chunks of information. You may want to use the table of contents and the chapter headings as a way to organize your thoughts about what you have learned and what you want to begin incorporating into your daily life. It may be helpful to create an annotated outline—an outline that includes your notes about what you have learned—and include the ways each chapter relates to your unique situation and your child.

In this chapter I will summarize what it is important to begin to think about regulating, how to identify where to begin, and finally if you are in the position to help others, how to be the best support. Let's begin by reviewing the key areas of regulation that were discussed in the second section of this book.

WHAT TO REGULATE

Environment

The environment is the first of the essential components consisting of the physical, temporal, and social environments. These three types of environments that your child experiences on a daily basis can be monitored, adjusted, and set to optimum levels and rhythms to ensure they are functioning at their best. I recommend that you begin by examining each of these environmental components relative to how well your child is doing in these areas.

Start with the routine physical environments that your child encounters on a daily basis. How is your child affected by them? Are there things that you need to change or adjust to help your child function better? If so, make note of the changes you make or would like to make over time. You can then move on to think about the activities and experiences your child engages in on a daily or weekly basis. Are these well organized? Do they promote a sense of order and calmness for your child? Are the teaching strategies at your child's school promoting skills needed for lifelong learning? Teaching strategies might include having the child journal or learn to self-sequence events. Make note of the activities that your child does well with, and conversely, note the activities or strategies that they struggle with. Lastly, you should examine your child's social environment. Are those around your child positive and supportive? Do they understand the unique needs of your child? Does your child have at least one friend? Does your child feel safe in the social environment? These are the basic questions to begin with. Again, make a note of your answers to these questions. These will begin to guide your intervention strategies.

Eating and nutrition

The second and third components are eating and nutritional components, which are important for internal health and regulation of the body and brain. The foods your child eats, along with the quantities of each food, can be regulated on a daily basis to affect optimal functioning. You should begin by logging all the food and beverages that your child consumes on a daily basis. Is your child eating too much sugar, or processed or fast foods? Are foods used as rewards on a regular basis in your child's school or at home? Is your child below or above their recommended body weight? These are the fundamental food and eating questions to ask. Once you have these answers, write them down. Then, you can begin to think about what you might want to add or change. Remember, this book stresses the additive theory. If you child eats mostly processed foods, then you want to start to add whole foods without taking away the processed foods at first. It is also highly recommended that you learn simple cooking skills, which have been outlined in Chapter 5.

Emotional self-regulation

The fourth element is emotional self-regulation, which controls the functioning of the brain's emotions and reactions. There are many strategies that can be employed to keep the brain and body in a state of equilibrium for optimal functioning. As you review Chapter 6 you will find many strategies to help your child manage their stress by calming their body and mind. Does your child have any successful strategies that they currently use? Do you have a friend or anyone local who can help teach strategies to your child such as yoga, deep breathing, or music therapy? Do you have any strategies that you use now that you can teach to your child? Remember, just the act of going to a park or outside in nature can help reduce stress and promote emotional self-regulation. Make note of what you are currently doing. The more strategies you have, and the more frequently you practice these strategies, the better.

Energy

Energy regulation is the final essential element and can be controlled through just the right amount of exercise, sleep, and keeping a consistent daily rhythm. The body and brain love and crave consistency. Do you and your child get at least one hour of exercise a day? Is your child able to sleep through the night, getting at least eight hours of restful sleep? Do you have a set daily routine in terms of when you wake up, eat, go to the bathroom, and go to sleep? Start by answering these questions taking note of the most problematic areas. I would begin by creating time in your day to exercise, which can positively affect sleep and routine functioning. Remember, exercise is good for the whole family and can be fun. Start with just dancing in your living room or moving to music like Zumba while you cook or wash the dishes. Moving to fast-paced rhythmic music will increase the heart rate.

Summary of the four components

When these four components are brought together in harmony, regulated to achieve maximum functioning, you have the potential to change the outcome for your child. But, just like the tug boat, you must adjust these functions—sometimes on a day-to-day basis depending on the task at hand or the conditions of the environment. The good news is that now you are aware of what's working and what's not, you're on a path to success.

WHERE TO BEGIN

You cannot and should not feel pressured to change everything at once. The information provided in this book is meant to help and not add stress to your life. Change can happen gradually, which will be healthier for your child and for you. Every small change can be a positive one. Consult with others, and if possible, consult with your child in determining where to start. The most important thing to realize is that this is a lifestyle approach and should not feel like a burden.

Non-negotiables

I recommend beginning by prioritizing the most important element in your and your child's life that needs regulating. These elements are called the non-negotiables—basic principles or problems that you are committed to. For instance, when I first started learning about healthy foods, one of my non-negotiables was that I wanted my family to eat healthier. I knew, however, that cutting out fast foods like French fries might be difficult. These foods are addictive and sometimes hard to stop eating all at once. I learned that I could begin to substitute the fast food fries with my own healthy version as described in Chapter 5 and found at the end of the book in the recipe section. Even if it was just once a week to start with, this was a step in the right direction toward my goal of healthier eating.

Let's say you commit to giving up processed chicken nuggets, a favorite children's food. You would need to commit to making your own nuggets on the weekend. If you have a chef friend, they could help by preparing these healthy nuggets for you and your family. You may even need to avoid the temptation of stopping at the fast food restaurant by choosing another route to and from your home. You might want to carry the nuggets you made with you in your car, and have your child eat them before you pass by the fast food restaurant. In this way, you satisfy the craving before it arises.

The point is that you must find a way to change an established habit. The shift requires thought, strategy, and commitment, but it doesn't have to be difficult. It can actually be fun if you turn it into a detective game. Children with autism often like these types of games. Your whole family can weigh in on spotting problems, identifying positives, and coming up with ways to create change for the better.

My second non-negotiable was to increase the amount of exercise my family was getting. Exercise is critical to reducing stress. Like many families, our family stress was high. Since exercise goals are really hard to keep, I set my first goal at the minimum level of exercise. We started with walking the dog together for 20 minutes a day. Part of that walk included jogging on the spot to get our heart rates up. Everyone bought into this, and the dog, who also needed to get in shape, enjoyed the family walk.

To recap, two non-negotiables were to eat healthier foods and to exercise more. I started my program by being mindful of these two activities each day, and I observed the results closely. These were small steps. However, after one month, we all agreed that we felt better and had a positive feeling of accomplishment, which led to adding more goals and non-negotiables.

You can begin by identifying your own non-negotiables, but don't try to take on more than you can. Your initial list of non-negotiables may be long, but the energy you have to make change is most likely limited. You may just want to think about the after school or before bedtime routines. Or you may want to examine the physical environment and maximize and organize the space for better functioning. Whatever you choose, focus on your choice and commit to it.

Wake up in the morning problem

A good way to decide how to prioritize what is most important to you can often be found in the early morning hours after your brain is rested. I call this your "wake up in the morning" problem. This is a technique I learned while studying to be a health coach. The first thought that comes to mind when you wake up will likely be the element of your life you most want to change. It is typically something that is bothering you that lingers on your mind.

For example, I was working with a mother who told me that every morning she woke up thinking about whether her son would ever have a friend. She worried that he would be isolated for the rest of his life, as he struggled to engage with other children his age. His sister has many friends. While they are nice to her brother, they are not his friends. This was where this parent needed to focus. She needed a strategy to begin to help her son.

We talked about setting up a meeting with her child's teacher and asking for recommendations of who she might be able to pair her son with to begin to work on a friendship. The teacher was very willing to help and began pairing this child with another boy who was shy and also without a friend. At first, she supervised the boys and had them build Lego structures together. Once they got to know each other a little better, the mothers arranged for a play date. They made cookies and had fun with making animals out of vegetables. This was the beginning of a friendship. Remember, it only takes one friend to change a child's outlook.

When you wake up in the morning, write down your thoughts about what is bothering you the most. After a week or so, see if the problem is the same. Begin with this problem. Seek help if needed, and develop a plan that can positively affect this problem.

COACHING

Among the other roles I play in helping children who have autism, I am a certified integrative nutrition health coach. A health coach can be very helpful to families by creating and encouraging situations that support change. A health coach can empower parents to learn the skills necessary for lifestyle changes. As you read in the first section of this book, there are many roles that a coach can play, from teaching basic cooking techniques to calming the brain and body. A health coach for autism is someone with a broad base of knowledge that includes knowledge about autism, the effects of stress on a person with autism, and strategies for better health and lifestyle change.

If you wish to help a parent of a child with autism, there are a few techniques you must master, in addition to understanding the fundamentals in this book. A coach must master the art of listening. That is, you must allow the parent to do most of the talking. You are there to listen and understand the parent's problems or concerns. In order to make sure you interpreting their concerns, you must learn to ask open-ended questions. For example, if a parent says, "I'm exhausted every day," an open-ended question might be, "Why do you think that's so?" or "Can you tell me more about that?" These types of questions clarify and focus on what the parent is saying is the problem.

If you want to assist the parent, you have to understand what the problems are, and to what extent they are affecting the parent. A coach in this program should be looking for the problems that are the greatest source of stress. For example, if the parent's stress is caused by the child throwing temper tantrums, you need to first help the parent with strategies for self-relaxation. Then, you can work with the parent to explore the sources of the child's tantrums: lack of sleep, unstructured or confusing environments, physical pain or discomfort, and others.

A coach takes copious notes and observes the behavior of the parent as they talk. Oftentimes, body language gives further insights into how the parent is feeling. For example, if the parent keeps their arms crossed and close to their body and they are hunched over with little eye contact, this can signal that they are unsure or insecure about what to do. If they are comfortable and ready for change, then their body language may be more open. They may sit up tall, use arm or hand gestures while talking, and make consistent eye contact. These are generalizations, but they are helpful to think about as you learn to pay attention to the parent as they talk.

The use of humor, even in difficult situations, is important as it breaks through stress and tension, which frees the mind to think. A good coach will listen first and then guide the parent to develop manageable step-by-step goals. Parents frequently attempt to take on too much at once. This is where a coach can be very helpful. Keep the goal(s) simple and achievable. A coach should be available to check in at least once a week, providing resources and support. It's important that the parent knows that the coach is available. I would encourage you, though, to set limits about when you, the coach, are available. You must take care of yourself as well. A coach must know when to seek help from a professional if problems arise that need further expertise.

We have developed a very supportive coaching program for parents, educators, and other school-based professionals. Coaches are not able to provide medical or clinical interventions, but they can help you formulate the right questions to ask the professionals and provide support to you as you learn to the make changes that can lead to a happier and healthier life for you and your child.

SUMMARY

This book has been written to enlighten parents and others who support children with autism to look beyond the core features of autism and to recognize that stress has a major impact on children's day-to-day functioning. It is meant to be a foundational book with information, techniques, and strategies which restore the child's health so that learning can occur. Children cannot learn when they are under extreme stress, and many children with autism experience unusually high levels of stress. It is up to you as a parent or supporter to choose the information that will be most useful to your child. Not everything in this book will meet every child and family's needs, but hopefully it will set the stage to find solutions to help make everyone's life easier. Each child and family who receives help makes a difference because their lives are better—this book is meant to help.

EPILOGUE

About The Center for Discovery

The Center for Discovery, Inc., founded in 1948, is highly regarded and well established as a Center of Excellence in the evaluation and treatment of those with complex disabilities. It is a not-for-profit, nationally- and internationally-known provider of educational, health, and residential services for children and adults with complex disabilities and medical frailties, including an ever-growing number of individuals with ASD.

The Center provides integrated diagnostic, educational, clinical, medical, social, recreational, and creative arts programs that promote health, happiness, vitality, and daily living skills. The main program at The Center is located in Sullivan County, 90 minutes northwest of New York City. The program also operates an assessment and evaluation clinic in Manhattan.

The Center for Discovery manages the healthcare of some of the most medically complex and behaviorally challenged individuals in the US. The program operates a Department of Health Article 28 Diagnostic and Treatment Clinic, which is an NCQA Level III Patient Centered Medical Home, providing the highest level of care coordination, including medical and behavioral health services.

Over the past decade, The Center has created a groundbreaking interdisciplinary research program focused on developing a variety of methods and technologies to assess and document intervention efficacy to improve the medical and behavioral status of individuals with complex conditions including ASD. Utilizing its own expertise and that of its partner researchers from Harvard University, Georgia Institute of Technology,

Columbia University, New York University, the University of North Carolina, and others, The Center for Discovery is pioneering studies designed to improve and empirically validate a variety of supports for individuals and families impacted by significant developmental disabilities. The Center for Discovery is considered a leader in the provision of innovative services and pioneering research.

RECIPES FOR NON-TOXIC CLEANERS USING NATURAL INGREDIENTS

What you will need on hand as core ingredients for cleaning:

White distilled vinegar

Liquid castille soap

Salt

Lime or lemon (scent any
cleaners with these)

Borax[1]

Baking soda

Tea tree oil or lavender

Hydrogen peroxide

Kitchen and bathrooms: all-purpose cleaner

2 cups of water

3 tsp of liquid castille soap

1 tsp of tea tree oil

Mix all ingredients together and use a sponge or cloth to clean. You can store leftover cleaner in a bottle in a locked cabinet. I suggest storing all cleaners, including bars of soap, in places that are child proof.

Toilet bowl

1 cup of borax or baking soda

Allow to soak in toilet overnight, and then scrub and flush.

Glass and mirrors

1/3 cup of white distilled
vinegar

1 quart of water—room
temperature

Mix together and spray on glass surface. Use newspaper or paper bag to remove dirt/scum.

---

1   Borax, also known as sodium tetraborate, and is a boron mineral and salt that's mined directly from the ground. Borax *is not boric acid*.

Laundry and cutting boards: sanitizing and killing mold and mildew

Hydrogen peroxide   *Tea tree oil or lavender*

Add half a cup of hydrogen peroxide in lieu of bleach to remove stains in laundry.

Use an eighth of cup of hydrogen peroxide on a wet sponge to disinfect surfaces and kill mold.

Add one teaspoon of tea tree oil or lavender to two cups of water to kill mold and disinfect surfaces.

Air freshener or carpet deodorizer

Baking soda

Open box of baking soda and leave out to freshen air.

Sprinkle baking soda on carpet to remove odors.

Floors

¼ cup of castille soap   *2 gallons of warm water*
½ cup of white vinegar

Mix ingredients in large bucket and mop with sponge mop. You can add 10 to 20 drops of tea tree oil or lavender if you need an antiseptic.

Oven

1 small box of baking soda

Sprinkle baking soda on bottom of oven and spray with water; re-spray with water if it becomes dry. Allow to sit overnight then scoop up baking soda and rise very well with water until clean.

For the dog: flea powder

½ teaspoon of each dried   *¼ cup of cornstarch*
eucalyptus, rosemary and
pennyroyal

Mix together and sprinkle on dog's hair—always avoid face/eyes/nose/mouth.

BRISTOL STOOL CHART

THE BRISTOL STOOL FORM SCALE

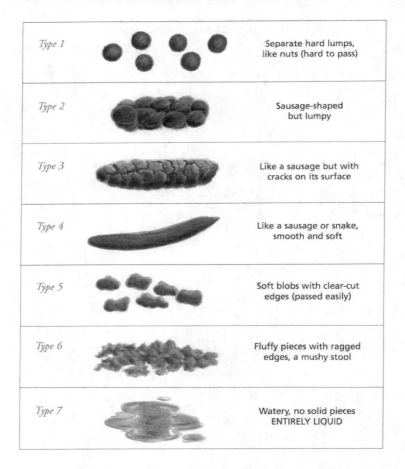

Type 1	Separate hard lumps, like nuts (hard to pass)
Type 2	Sausage-shaped but lumpy
Type 3	Like a sausage but with cracks on its surface
Type 4	Like a sausage or snake, smooth and soft
Type 5	Soft blobs with clear-cut edges (passed easily)
Type 6	Fluffy pieces with ragged edges, a mushy stool
Type 7	Watery, no solid pieces ENTIRELY LIQUID

Reproduced with kind permission of Dr KW Heaton, formerly Reader in Medicine at the University of Bristol. ©2000, Norgine group of companies.

RECIPES

RANCH IN A JAR

Who doesn't love to dip their veggies in ranch? This recipe is fun for kids to make and helps with tasting and trying new vegetables.

Yield 2½ cups
Portion size 1 tbsp
Number of portions 40

1 cup mayonnaise

1 cup plain whole yogurt

½ cup whole sour cream

1 tsp garlic powder

1 tsp onion powder

1 tbsp granulated sugar

1 tbsp rice vinegar
unseasoned, optional

1 tsp salt

1 tbsp dried parsley

Place all ingredients into a 1-quart mason jar with a tight-fitting lid. Screw lid on tightly and shake until all ingredients are mixed. Store in refrigerator for up to one week.

CAULIFLOWER CRUST PIZZA

A gluten free way to serve a favorite and get some much needed vegetables into the mix!

Serves 2; Adapted from Your Lighter Side

1 cup cooked, riced cauliflower

1 cup shredded mozzarella cheese

1 egg, beaten

1 tsp dried oregano

½ tsp crushed garlic

½ tsp garlic salt

olive oil (optional)

Pizza sauce, shredded cheese and your choice of toppings[1]

To "rice" the cauliflower:

1. Take one large head of fresh cauliflower, remove stems and leaves, and chop the florets into chunks.

2. Add to food processor and pulse until it looks like grain. Do not over-do pulse or you will puree it. (If you don't have a food processor, you can grate the whole head with a cheese grater).

3. Place the riced cauliflower into a microwave safe bowl and microwave for eight minutes (some microwaves are more powerful than others, so you may need to reduce this cooking time). There is no need to add water, as the natural moisture in the cauliflower is enough to cook itself.

One large head should produce approximately three cups of riced cauliflower. The remainder can be used to make additional pizza crusts immediately, or can be stored in the refrigerator for up to one week.

To make the pizza crust:

1. Preheat oven to 230°C/450°F. Spray a cookie sheet with non-stick cooking spray.

2. In a medium bowl, stir together 1 cup riced cauliflower, the beaten egg and the mozzarella. Add oregano, crushed garlic and garlic salt then stir.

3. Transfer to the cookie sheet, and using your hands, pat out into a 9" round. Optional: brush olive oil over top of mixture to help with browning.

---

1   Note that toppings need to be precooked since you are only broiling for a few minutes.

4. Bake for 15 minutes.

5. Remove from oven. To the crust, add sauce, toppings, and cheese. Place under a broiler at high heat just until cheese is melted (approximately 3–4 minutes).

BANANA CHOCO-CHIP MUFFINS

These are a protein packed breakfast or snack that most kids love. One of our favorite recipes!

Yield 6
Portion size 1
Number of portions 6

1 cup almond meal flour
1/4 cup coconut flour
1/4 cup chocolate chips
1/4 cup sea salt
1/2 tsp baking soda
1/4 tsp baking powder

1 tbsp honey
1 fl oz coconut oil
1 1/2 large eggs
1 1/2 tsp pure vanilla extract
2/3 cup banana, ripe, mashed

1. Preheat oven to 180°C/350°F.

2. In a mixing bowl, combine all dry ingredients—almond meal four, coconut flour, chocolate chips, salt, baking soda, and baking powder.

3. In a separate mixing bowl, combine wet ingredients except banana—honey, eggs, coconut oil (melted over a very low flame or microwave) and vanilla.

4. Add the wet ingredients to the dry and combine until smooth. Fold in mashed banana.

5. Line a 6 cup muffin pan with paper liners. Using a 1/4 cup measure, scoop batter into the muffin cups.

6. Place in the preheated oven and bake for 20–25 minutes until tops are golden brown. (Note: These muffins do not rise like typical flour muffins.)

TRADITIONAL CHICKEN FINGERS

This recipe works to transition off of fast food chicken nuggets. The chicken can be cut into either strips or nuggets depending on preference.

Yield 24 pieces
Portion size 4 oz
Number of portions 6

1 ½ lb boneless skinless chicken breast 4 oz each

⅓ cup all-purpose unbleached flour

3 large eggs

¾ cup plain bread crumbs

1. Preheat oven to 200°C/400°F.
2. Trim each chicken breast of any fat.
3. Pound each into an even thinness, about ½ inch.
4. Slice each chicken breast into about four even strips.
5. Place flour, eggs, and bread crumbs in three separate shallow containers.
6. Coat each piece of chicken with flour, dip in egg, then in bread crumbs to coat each side. Continue until all chicken is coated.
7. Lightly oil sheet pan and preheat in oven for 3–5 minutes.
8. Place pieces on a lightly oiled baking sheet.
9. Bake for 15 minutes, turning once, until internal temperature reaches 165°C/320°F.

FAST FOOD FRIES

This is an easy recipe to mimic your child's favorite fast food fries. You can even put them in a paper bag initially to give the same experience that your child is used to. Once these fries are accepted, use sweet potato or zucchini for variety.

Yield 2 lbs
Serving size ¼ lb
Number of portions 8

2 lb potato russet/baking potato

sea salt

¼ tsp high oleic sunflower oil (if not found, sunflower, peanut or avocado oil works)

1. Wash and peel potatoes if desired.
2. Cut potatoes into fry shape using a French fry press, or hand cut.
3. Rinse potatoes after cutting. If necessary, store potatoes in fresh water overnight.
4. Drain.
5. Heat frying pan on medium high heat. Fill to 1 inch deep with oil. Allow oil to rise to temperature (small bubbles should be apparent).
6. Place single layer of fries in oil.
7. Cook fries turning on occasion until fry becomes opaque before potato starts browning.
8. Lift fries out of oil and place on paper towel to absorb some oil.
9. Then place in single layer on parchment lined sheet pans.
10. Freeze. Once frozen store in bulk container in freezer.

At service:

1. Repeat above frying technique and cook fries in oil until golden brown color.
2. Lift fries out of oil and place on paper towel.
3. Sprinkle with sea salt and serve.

FARMER'S MACARONI AND CHEESE

A great way to incorporate veggies into a kid favorite! The ratio of pasta to vegetable can change as your child becomes more accepting of the vegetable. We like cauliflower to start because it appears similar to the pasta in terms of color but any vegetable can be substituted.

Yield hotel pan (12x24, 2" deep)
Number of portions 12

4 lbs fresh cauliflower, cut into florets

1 lb penne, wholewheat pasta

2 gallons water, boiling

1 tbsp sea salt

1 tbsp olive, extra virgin oil

6 oz salted butter

4 oz all-purpose unbleached flour

½ tbsp mustard, dry spice

1 oz Worcestershire sauce

2 quarts whole milk

2 lbs wedge cheese, grated

For topping:

1 lb fresh bread crumbs

1 tsp thyme, fresh herb, leaf only

3 oz salted butter, melted

1. Preheat oven to 180°C/350°F. Butter hotel pan.
2. Bring a large pot of salted water to a boil. Add the cauliflower and cook for six minutes. Lift out of the water with a strainer.
3. Add pasta to the same water and cook until just barely tender. Drain.
4. Toss cauliflower and pasta with olive oil. Set aside.
5. Make the cheese sauce: make a white roux—melt the butter, stir in the flour, salt and dry mustard. Cook for 5–10 minutes. Do not allow to brown.
6. Add milk, stirring constantly with a whisk. Cook until mixture comes to a simmer and thickens.
7. Add cheese to sauce. Stir until cheese melts and is incorporated. Stir in Worcestershire sauce. Mix in cauliflower and pasta.

8. Scale into buttered half hotel pan—6 lbs per pan—12 servings per pan.

9. Mix bread crumbs, thyme, and melted butter. Sprinkle over the macaroni and cheese.

10. Bake in oven at 180°C/ 350°F until the edges bubble and the top is light brown (approximately 10 minutes).

BLACK BEAN BROWNIES

Black bean brownies are gluten free and require just one bowl and about 30 minutes to prepare! Healthy, easy and delicious— the best kind of dessert!

Yield 12
Portion size 1
Number of portions 12

1 15 oz can black beans, well rinsed and drained (around 1 ¾ cups)

2 large egg

3 tbsp coconut oil, melted (or butter)

¾ cup cocoa powder (the higher quality the better)

¼ tsp sea salt

1 tsp pure vanilla extract

½ cup raw sugar, slightly ground or pulsed in a food processor or coffee grinder for refined texture

1 ½ tsp baking powder

Optional toppings: crushed walnuts, pecans or semisweet chocolate chips

1. Preheat oven to 180°C/350°F.

2. Lightly grease a 12-slot standard size muffin pan (not mini). Make sure you've rinsed and thoroughly drained your black beans at this point.

3. Add all ingredients (besides walnuts or other toppings) and puree—about three minutes—scraping down sides as needed. It should be fairly smooth. If the batter appears too thick, add a

tbsp or two of water and pulse again. It should be slightly less thick than chocolate frosting but nowhere close to runny.

4. Evenly distribute the batter into the muffin tin and smooth the tops with a spoon or your finger. Optional: Sprinkle with crushed walnuts, pecans or chocolate chips.

5. Bake for 20–25 minutes or until the tops are dry and the edges start to pull away from the sides.

6. Remove from oven and let cool for 30 minutes before removing from the pan.

7. They will be tender, so remove gently with a fork. The insides are meant to be very fudgy, so don't be concerned if they seem too moist—that's the point.

8. Store in an airtight container for up to a few days. Refrigerate to keep longer.

CHOCOLATE PUDDING

Yield 6 cups
Portion ½ cup
Number of portions 12

1 cup granulated sugar

4 tbsp cornstarch

½ cup cocoa powder

¼ tsp sea salt

12 egg yolks

2 ½ cups whole milk

2 ½ cups heavy cream

2 tsp organic vanilla extract

8 oz dark chocolate, chopped

Whipping cream for garnish

1. Sift sugar, cornstarch, cocoa powder and salt together into a large mixing bowl.

2. Add the egg yolks and whisk until well combined. Set aside.

3. In a medium-sized, heavy-bottomed sauce pot, bring the milk, cream, and vanilla extract to a boil.

4. Working quickly, pour the milk over the egg mixture and whisk until combined.

5. Return the mixture to the sauce pot and bring the mixture to a boil, over medium heat.

6. When the mixture has bubbled, pass it through a fine-mesh strainer and back into the mixing bowl.

7. Add the chocolate. Whisk until well combined.

8. Gently press a layer of plastic wrap onto the surface of the pudding and chill.

9. Refrigerate until needed.

10. Transfer to dessert cups and finish with a dollop of whipped cream before serving.

CHOCOLATE PUDDING, AVOCADO

A yummy treat that isn't all that it seems. Best if made and eaten immediately.

Yield 1 ½ cups
Portion size ½ cup
Number of portions 3

1 avocado
¼ cup cocoa powder, dark unsweetened

¼ cup honey
1 tsp vanilla extract

Place avocado, cocoa powder, honey, and vanilla into a food processor and blend until smooth.

A small amount of water may be needed in order to get the desired consistency (1–4 tbsp).

Note: The size of the avocado may alter the quantities of the cocoa powder and honey needed. Adjust these to taste.

HARVEST MEATLOAF

Incorporating vegetables into a more traditional dish can be a great way to minimize the focus of vegetables on a plate. But remember it's very important not to hide foods or mislead kids about ingredients. It works best not to highlight the vegetable and instead move it inside a well-accepted dish.

Yield 1 meatloaf
Portion size 1 slice
Number of portions 6

2 tbsp extra virgin olive oil

¾ cup finely chopped spring onion

2 cloves garlic, minced

¾ cup finely diced celery

½ cup peeled and grated broccoli stalk

1 cup grated sweet potato

2 lbs ground 90 percent lean beef

1 can tomato paste

1 cup cooked basmati brown rice

2 large eggs, slightly beaten

1 tbsp Worcestershire sauce

1 tbsp chopped chives

1 tsp salt

¼ tsp freshly ground black pepper

1 ½ tsp dry mustard

½ cup ketchup

1. Preheat the oven to 180°C/350°F.
2. Place the olive oil in a sauté pan with the spring onion, garlic, celery, broccoli stalk, and sweet potato.
3. Heat over medium until the vegetables are soft but not brown.
4. Remove from heat and cool.
5. In a large bowl, combine ground beef, tomato paste, cooked brown rice, the cooled, cooked vegetables, egg, Worcestershire sauce, thyme, chives, dry mustard, and pepper. Mix lightly but thoroughly.
6. Shape the mixture into a loaf approximately 9" long x 4" wide x 3" high.

7. Place on a baking pan lined with foil. Top with ketchup.
8. Bake in the oven for 45 minutes to 1 hour or until no longer pink and juices run clear, 165°C/320°F internal temperature.
9. Cut each meat loaf into six equal portions, approximately 1½" thick.

MATT'S ALMOND COOKIES

This "cookie" packs a protein and healthy fat punch. We use this cookie for dessert with a meal we aren't sure will be readily accepted. The cookie ensures good nutrition while working with transition foods.

Yield 20
Portion size 2
Number of portions 10

¼ cup coconut oil, melted (or softened butter)

¼ cup honey

2 large eggs

2 tsp vanilla, pure extract

1 tsp baking soda

¼ tsp salt

3 cups almond meal flour

1 cup shredded unsweetened coconut

1. Preheat oven to 140°C/275°F.
2. Combine all ingredients, adding almond flour and coconut last.
3. Form dough into balls.
4. Place on buttered baking sheet and flatten.
5. Bake in preheated oven for about 15 minutes or until golden around the edges.

For variety, add ½—1 cup chocolate chips or roll balls in a dish of cinnamon sugar before baking. The dough can be frozen to have fresh baked cookies on hand at almost any time!

GLUTEN-FREE CHICKEN NUGGETS

This chicken nugget recipe is the definition of easy. This is a gluten-free option that most kids love. I recommend using the other chicken finger recipe if your child likes to eat the breading off their nuggets to start and then move them to this version. The arrowroot adheres well to the chicken but will not create a very thick crust.

Yield 24
Portion size 4–6 nuggets
Number of portions 4

Boneless, skinless chicken breast

Arrowroot powder (flour)

Ghee (clarified butter)

Salt

1. Trim chicken breast and cut into 2" chunks—nugget sized.
2. Pour arrowroot powder on a plate.
3. Dredge chicken chunks in arrowroot until covered on all sides (arrowroot adheres very well).
4. Heat a pan (or a wok works well) with ghee on medium heat. (Ghee should be deep enough that when nuggets are added the ghee comes half way up the nugget.)
5. Fry nuggets in ghee on each side until chicken is cooked in the center and the outside is light brown.
6. Lay cooked nuggets on paper towel to absorb excess ghee.
7. Sprinkle with a coarse salt while still hot. Serve.

THE ABCS OF ENERGYM AEROBIC, BALANCE, CORE, COORDINATION, STRENGTHENING

AEROBIC
Bounce disc

Muscles targeted: heart, legs and glutes
Benefits: increased cardiovascular endurance

1. Begin standing on top of bounce pad.
2. Jump 50–100 times before taking a break.
3. Repeat.

Jogging on BOSU, on the spot, or on a treadmill

Muscles targeted: total body and core
Benefits: balance training as well as increased cardiovascular endurance

Jumping jacks

Muscles targeted: legs, shoulders, core
Benefits: increased cardiovascular endurance, coordination and the promotion of motor planning ability

1. Stand with feet together and arms at sides.
2. Jump while raising arms and separating legs to sides, land with arms overhead and legs apart.
3. Repeat 10 times.

Burpees

Muscles targeted: total body
Benefits: increased endurance

1. Stand up straight, then get into a squat position with your hands on the floor in front of you.
2. Kick your feet back into a push up position and immediately drop your chest to the ground.
3. Bow your chest up, then return your feet back to the squat position as fast as possible.
4. Immediately jump up into the air as high as you can.
5. You can add a clap at the end.
6. Repeat 10 times.

Step-ups

Muscles targeted: heart, legs, and glutes
Benefits: increased cardiovascular endurance, muscular strength and endurance, balance, motor planning

1. Stand in front of step, low bench, stair or other solid surface about 8 to 10 inches high.
2. Step up with right leg (lead leg).
3. Bring left leg up to meet right.
4. Bring left leg down to floor.
5. Bring right leg down to floor.
6. Repeat 20–30 times then repeat with left leg as the lead.

BALANCE
One leg

Muscles targeted: legs, feet, ankles, and core
Benefits: increased stability, balance

1. Stand with feet shoulder-width apart.
2. Lift right leg up as though you are stepping.
3. Bring right foot up to left inner side of knee.
4. Hold to pose for one minute or as long as you can while maintaining your balance.
5. Switch to left leg after five consecutive trials.
6. Build up strength to hold up to three minutes with each leg.

BOSU ball activities
Standing mountain pose

Muscles targeted: legs, feet, ankles, core
Benefits: increased stability, balance

1. Stand on the floor behind the dome with good posture, hands down at sides.
2. Place one foot on top of the dome.
3. Step up on dome to a centered position.
4. Hold this balanced position for 10–60 seconds.
5. Step down to floor back to starting position.
6. Repeat 10 times.

Standing mountain pose with arm movements

Muscles targeted: legs, feet, ankles, core
Benefits: increase stability, balance

While standing on BOSU perform various arm movements for increased challenge

1. Outstretch arms overhead, place arms to sides—repeat 10 times.
2. Arm circles—circle arms to sides 10 times.
3. Name various body parts and have student/child touch with hand(s):
    I. top of head
    II. eyes
    III. nose
    IV. mouth
    V. chin
    VI. shoulders
    VII. stomach
    VIII. knees
    IX. feet.

Dome squat

Muscles targeted: legs, feet and ankles, core
Benefits: balance, muscular strength and endurance

1. Stand centered on the top of the dome, feet hip-width apart.
2. Slowly bend at the hips, knees and ankles.
3. Picture yourself sitting in a chair.
4. Do not allow knees to go past the tips of your toes.
5. Allow arms to reach forward to counterbalance the backward motion of the hips.
6. Pause.
7. Then slowly return to starting position.

Jump and stick

> **Muscles targeted:** legs, feet, ankle, core
> **Benefits:** balance, muscular strength and endurance, coordination

1. While standing centered on the BOSU (bend knees, elbows bent).
2. Jump straight up.
3. Land in center of BOSU.
4. Hold in place for 2–3 seconds.
5. Repeat 10 times.

30 inch fitness ball activities — sitting
Sitting on a fitness ball

> **Muscles targeted:** core (trunk control and postural control)
> **Benefits:** balance, muscular strength

How to sit on a fitness ball

1. Sit in the center of the ball with feet in front of the ball on the floor.
2. Feet and knees should be facing forward.
3. Feet and knees should be hip-width apart.
4. Prompt student/child to sit as straight as possible—cues may include sit tall, chin in, shoulders back.

Basic arm movements while sitting on a fitness ball

Muscles targeted: core (trunk control and postural control), shoulders, back
Benefits: balance, muscular strength, motor planning, coordination

1. Sit on ball (see above).
2. Raise both arms to sides of body until even with shoulders.
3. Hold, lower arms, and repeat.

Variation:
Arms overhead: raise both arms to sides of body until hands are directly overhead.

Knee raises while sitting on a fitness ball

Muscles targeted: core, legs
Benefits: balance, muscular strength, motor planning, coordination

1. Sit on ball (see above).
2. Lift right knee toward chest, bringing right foot from floor.
3. Hold, then return right foot to floor.
4. Repeat with left foot.
5. Continue to alternate feet.

Unilateral arms and legs while sitting on a fitness ball

> **Muscles targeted:** core, legs, arms
> **Benefits:** balance, muscular strength, motor planning, coordination

1. Sit on ball (see above).
2. Extend right leg forward and slightly to side while also lifting right arm up and slightly to side.
3. Return to starting position.
4. Extend left leg forward and slightly to side while also lifting left arm up and slightly to side.
5. Return to starting position.
6. Repeat these alternating sides.

Balance beam/ tape line
Walking forward on a balance beam/tape line

> **Muscles targeted:** legs, core
> **Benefits:** balance, motor planning, coordination

1. Start by placing one foot on the beam/line.
2. Next place second foot in front of the first, keeping in mind to place entire foot on beam for stability.
3. Prompt student/child to look down at the beam/tape.
4. Hold arms out to sides like an airplane.
5. Continue putting one foot in front of the other while walking on the beam/tape.

Walking backwards on a balance beam/tape line

1. Start by placing one foot on the beam/line backwards.
2. Next place second foot behind the first, keeping in mind to place entire foot on beam for stability.
3. Prompt student/child to look down at the beam/tape.
4. Hold arms out to sides like an airplane.
5. Continue putting one foot behind of other while walking on the beam/tape.

Walking sideways on a balance beam tape line

1. Start by standing with both feet perpendicular on the beam/tape.
2. The center of the foot should be used to contact the beam/tape for optimal stability.
3. Hold arms out to sides like an airplane.
4. Start moving down the beam sideways, one foot leading the other.

CORE
Crunches on BOSU

Muscles targeted: core, hip, and shoulder stabilization
Benefits: balance, muscular strength and endurance, motor planning

1. Lie on your back on the dome side of BOSU—your lower back should be centered on the dome.
2. Position feet on the floor about shoulder-width apart.
3. Cross hands over chest.
4. Gently pull your abs inward curling up and forward 2–3 inches.
5. Shoulder blades rise off the BOSU.
6. Gently lower to starting position.
7. Repeat 10 times.

Crunches on mat

> **Muscles targeted:** stomach and back
> **Benefits:** strengthening, better posture in sitting and standing

1. Lie on your back on mat.
2. Position feet on the floor about shoulder width apart.
3. Cross hands over chest.
4. Gently pull your abs inward curling up and forward 2–3 inches.
5. Shoulder blades rise off the mat.
6. Gently lower to starting position.
7. Repeat ten times.

COORDINATION

See earlier in section for:

Jumping jacks

Step-ups

Balance beam

STRENGTHENING (TOTAL BODY AND CORE)

Push up progression

> **Muscles targeted:** chest, back, stomach, shoulders, muscles at the back of your upper arm
> **Benefits:** strengthening these muscles will enhance the ability of your child to sit/stand in an upright position for extended periods of time without slouching or leaning on support surfaces

Wall push ups and elevated push ups are great exercises to practice in order to build your body up to be ready to perform a traditional push up.

Wall push up

1. Set your hands on the wall in front of you, slightly wider than shoulder-width apart.
2. Walk your feet backward until your elbows are fully extended and your arms are supporting your weight.
3. Envision your body as a straight line from head to toe (buttocks should not be swaying forward or backward).
4. Lower your body at a steady rate toward the wall (nose almost touching the wall).
5. Push back to your beginning position.

Elevated push ups (progression from wall push ups)

1. Choose a table-height surface.
2. Start position will be the same as for the wall push up (only difference being that your hands will be set on the table height surface rather than a wall).
3. Lower your body at a steady rate toward the elevated surface (nose almost touching elevated surface).
4. Push back to your beginning position.

Traditional push up

1. On a mat, set hands at a distance that is slightly wider than shoulder-width apart.
2. Position feet so that they are touching or as far as shoulder-width apart (the wider your feet, the more stable you will feel).
3. Envision your body as a straight line from head to toe (buttocks should not be pushed up or down).
4. Before beginning, tense your buttocks and stomach muscles in order to engage your core. This will provide more stability for you as you begin the exercise.

5. Lower your body at a steady rate until your elbows reach a 90-degree angle. (Some people may be able to lower themselves so that their elbows reach lower than 90 degrees.)

6. Once you have lowered your body, pause, and then push back up to your starting position.

Abdominal hip thrust

> **Muscles targeted:** core, legs
> **Benefits:** endurance, strengthening, motor planning

1. Lay on your back on a mat.
2. Bend your knees in order to place feet flat on the mat.
3. Look directly up.
4. Lift your hips and buttocks off the mat.
5. Slowly lower back down to the mat.
6. Repeat 10 times.

Single leg kickbacks

> **Muscles targeted:** core, buttocks, shoulders
> **Benefits:** strengthening, coordination, motor planning

1. Assume a hands and knees position on the mat.
2. Lift one leg up and off of the mat so that it is in line with your trunk (knee should be straight).
3. Slowly lower back to mat.
4. Repeat 10 times.
5. Follow same steps with opposite leg.

30 inch fitness ball activities—standing

Squat with a ball

Muscles targeted: thighs, hips, buttocks, quadriceps, hamstrings, back
Benefits: muscular endurance and strengthening, balance

1. Place fitness ball between wall and curve of your lower back.
2. Feet shoulder-width apart.
3. Bend knees and lower 5–10 inches. Make sure to keep shoulders level and hips square to ground.
4. Hold for 1–3 seconds.
5. Return to starting position.

Fitness ball roll on wall

Muscles targeted: shoulders, core
Benefits: muscular strength and endurance, motor planning

1. Find a clear wall space approximately 6 feet wide.
2. Place ball on wall over student/child's head.
3. Students/child's arms should be outstretched with ball able to be reached at students/child's hands.
4. Start at one end of the cleared wall space and roll the ball along wall hand over hand.
5. When you reach your stopping point, repeat in reverse direction.

Hand-held weight exercises
Bicep curls

> **Muscles targeted:** biceps
> **Benefits:** muscular strength and endurance

1. Stand up straight, legs shoulder-width apart.
2. Hold dumbbell in one hand. Make sure thumbs are curled around grips.
3. Hold dumbbell at sides—palms facing forward.
4. Bend elbows and slowly bring dumbbells to your chest.
5. Lower and repeat 10 times.
6. Switch hands and repeat exercise with opposite arm.

Lateral deltoid raise

> **Muscles targeted:** back (middle deltoids)
> **Benefits:** muscular strength and endurance

1. Hold dumbbell at the sides of the thighs.
2. With elbows slight bent, raise arms upward to the side until dumbbells are slightly higher than shoulder level.
3. Lower and repeat 10 times.

Shrugs

> **Muscles targeted:** back, shoulders
> **Benefits:** muscular strength and endurance

1. Stand, holding dumbbells alongside your thighs.
2. Elevate shoulders as high as possible.
3. Lower and repeat 10 times.

REFERENCES

Ahlskog, J.E., Geda, Y.E., Graff-Radford, N.R. and Petersen R.C. (2011) "Physical exercise as a preventive or disease-modifying treatment of dementia and brain aging." *Mayo Clinic Proceedings 86, 9,* 876.

Albeck, D.S., Kazuhiro, S., Gayle, E.P. and Dalton, L. (2006) "Mild forced treadmill exercise enhances spatial learning in the aged rat." *Behavior Brain Research 168, 2,* 345–348.

American Psychiatric Association (2013) *Diagnostic and Statistical Manual of Mental Disorders* (5th edn.). Washington, DC: APA.

Bandura, A. (1982) "Self-efficacy mechanism in human agency." *American Psychologist 37, 2,* 122-147.

Bandura, A. (1986) *Social Foundations of Thought and Action: A Social Cognitive Theory.* Upper Saddle River, NJ: Prentice Hall.

Bandura, A. (1993) "Perceived self-efficacy in cognitive development and functioning." *Educational Psychologist 28,* 117–148.

Bandura, A. (1997) *Self-Efficacy: The Exercise of Control.* New York: Freeman Publishers.

Baron-Cohen, S., Leslie, A.M. and Fitch, U. (1985) "Does the autistic child have theory of mind?" *Cognition 21,* 37–46.

Bassuk, S.S., Church, T.S. and Manson, J.E. (2013) "Why exercise works magic." *Scientific American Magazine 399, 2,* 79–89.

Bauman, M.L. and Kemper, T.L. (2005) "Neuroanatomic observations of the brain in autism: a review and future directions." *International Journal of Developmental Neuroscience 2, 23,* 183–187.

Beilock, S.L. (2015) *How The Body Knows Its Mind: The Surprising Power of the Physical Environment to Influence How You Think and Feel.* New York: Simon and Schuster.

Benson, D. and Donohoe, R.T. (1999) "The effects of nutrients on mood." *Public Health Nutrition 2,* 3A, 403–409.

Berger, N.I. and Ingersoll, B. (2013) "An exploration of imitation recognition in young children with autism spectrum disorders." *Autism Research, 6, 5,* 411–416.

Bergland, C. (2014) "Chronic Stress Can Damage Brain Structure and Connectivity Chronic stress and high levels of cortisol create long-lasting brain changes." *The Athletes Way.* Post, February 12.

Betts, D.E. and Betts, S.W. (2006) *Yoga for Children with Autism Spectrum Disorders: A Step by Step Guide for Parents and Caregivers.* London: Jessica Kingsley Publishers.

Bleuler, E. (1950) *Dementia Praecox or the Group of Schizophrenias*. New York: International Universities Press.

Bouchard, M.F., Bellinger, D.C., Wright, R.O. and Weisskopf, M.G. (2010) "Attention-deficit/hyperactivity disorder and urinary metabolites of organophosphate pesticides." *Pediatrics 125*, 6, 1270–1277.

Brand, S., Dunn, R. and Greb, F. (2002) "Learning styles of students with attention deficit hyperactivity disorder: who are they and how can we teach them?" *The Clearing House 75*, 5, 268–273.

Bresnahan, M., Hornig, M., Schultz, A.F., Guennes, N. *et al.* (2015) "Association of maternal report of infant and toddler gastrointestinal symptoms with autism." *JAMA Psychiatry 72*, 5, 466–474.

Broda, H.W. (2011) *Moving the Classroom Outdoors: Schoolyard Enhanced Learning in Action*. Portland, ME: Stenhouse Publishers.

Buie, T. (2015) *Autism Speaks Website: Acid Reflux Q&A with Autism- GI specialist Tim Buie*. Available at www.autismspeaks.org/science/science-news/office-hours-gi-specialist-tim-buie-acid-reflux-and-autism, accessed on 07 January, 2015.

Buie, T., Campbell, D.B., Fuchs, G.J., 3rd and Furuta, G.T. *et al.* (2010) "Recommendations for evaluation and treatment of common gastrointestinal problems in children with ASDs." *Pediatrics 125*, 1, 19–29.

Cautela, J.R. and Groden, J. (1978) *Relaxation: A Comprehensive Manual for Adults, Children, and Children with Special Needs*. Champaign, IL: Research Press.

Centers for Disease Control and Prevention Prevalence of autism spectrum disorder among children aged 8 years -autism and developmental disabilities monitoring network, 11 sites, United States, 2010. (2014) MMWR Surveill Summary, 63(Suppl2):1–21.

Chu, P., Gotink, R.A., Yeh, G.Y., Goldie, S.J. and Hunink, M.M. (2014) "The effectiveness of yoga in modifying risk factors for cardiovascular disease and metabolic syndrome: a systematic review and meta-analysis of randomized controlled trials." doi: 10.1177/2047487314562741.

Clements, R. (2004) "An investigation of the status of outdoor play." *Contemporary Issues in Early Childhood 5*, 68–80.

Corbett, B.A. and Simon, D. (2013) "Adolescence, stress and cortisol in autism spectrum disorders." *Open Access Autism 1*, 1, 2.

Corbett, B.A., Schupp, C.W., Levine, S. and Mendoza, S. (2009) "Comparing cortisol, stress and sensory stimulation in children with autism." *Autism Research: Official Journal of the International Society for Autism Research 2*, 1, 39–49.

Corbett, B.A., Schupp, C.W., Simon, D., Ryan, N. and Mendoza, S. (2010) "Elevated cortisol during play is associated with age and social engagement in children with autism." *Molecular Autism 1*, 13.

Courchesne, E., Mouton, P.R., Calhoun, M.E. and Semendeferi, K. *et al.* (2011) "Neuron number and size in prefrontal cortex of children with autism." *JAMA 11*, 18, 306.

Coury, D. (2010) "Medical treatment of autism spectrum disorders." *Current Opinion in Neurology 23*, 2, 131–136.

Croen, L. (2014) *Kaiser Permanente Northern California Division of Research, Oakland, California.* May 15, 2014. International Meeting for Autism Research: Atlanta, GA. Available at www.autismspeaks.org/science/science-news/adults-autism-suffer-high-rates-most-major-disorders, accessed on 07 January, 2015.

Curtin, C., Anderson, S.E., Must, A. and Bandini, L. (2010) "The prevalence of obesity in children with autism: a secondary analysis using nationally representative data from the National Survey of Children's Health." *Biomedical Central Pediatrics 10*, 11, 1–5.

Czerniak, C.M. and Chiarelott, L. (1990) "Teacher education for effective science instruction: a social cognitive perspective." *Journal of Teacher Education 41*, 1, 49–58.

Davidson, M.H., Hunninghake, D., Maki, K., Kwiterovich, P.O. and Kafonek, S. (1999) "Comparison of the effects of lean red meat vs. lean white meat on serum lipid levels among free-living persons with hypercholesterolemia: a long-term, randomized clinical trial." *Archives of Internal Medicine 159*, 12, 1331–1338.

Davies, M.M. (1996) "Outdoors: an important context for young children's development." *Early Child Development and Care 115*, 3749.

de Shazo, R.D., Bigler, S. and Baldwin-Skipworth, L. (2013) "The autopsy of chicken nuggets reads 'chicken little'." *The American Journal of Medicine 126*, 1018–1019.

Doidge, N. (2007) *The Brain that Changes Itself: Stories of Personal Triumph from the Frontiers of Brain Science.* New York: Viking.

Donnerstein, E. and Wilson, D.W. (1976) "Effects of noise and perceived control on ongoing and subsequent aggressive behavior." *Journal of Personality and Social Psychology 34*, 774–781.

Dufault, R., Lukiw, W., Crider, R. and Schnoll, R. *et al.* (2012) "A macro-epigenetic approach to identifying factors responsible for the autism epidemic in the United States." *Clinical Epigenetics 4*, 1, 6.

Dunn-Buron, K. and Curtis, M. (2012) *The Incredible 5-point Scale: The Significantly Improved and Expanded Second Edition.* Lenexa, KS: AAPC Publishing.

Dweck, C.S. (2000) *Self-theories: Their Role in Motivation, Personality, and Development.* Philadelphia, PA: Taylor and Francis.

Dzulkifli, M.A. and Mustafar, M.F. (2013) "The influence of colour on memory performance: a review." *Malays Journal of Medical Science 20*, 2, 3–9.

Easter Seals (2008) *Living with autism study: Harris Interactive/Easter Seals.* Available at http://es.easterseals.com/site/DocServer/Study_FINAL_ Harris_12.4.08_Compressed.pdf?docID=83143, accessed on 29 September, 2012.

Eckhardt, M., Ferguson, C. and Picard, R. (2013) *Story Scape: A project from the MIT Media Lab affective computing group.* Available at https://storyscape. io/about/, accessed on 22 January, 2015.

Elliot, A.J., Maier, M.A., Moller, A.C., Friedman, R. and Meinhardt, J. (2007) "Color and psychological functioning: the effect of red on performance attainment." *Journal of Experimental Psychology 136,* 1, 154–168.

Environmental Working Group, The (2015) *Shopper's Guide.* Available at http://www.ewg.org/foodnews/index.php, accessed on 15 March, 2015.

Fielding, R. (2006) "Best practice in action: six essential elements that define educational facility design." *The CEFPI Educational Facility Planner,* October 30, 1–7.

Fielding, R. (2009) "Designing personalized spaces that impact student achievement: a case study of Cristo Rey High School." *The CEFPI Educational Facility Planner 43,* 2&3, 33–37.

Fox, S. (1996) *Human Physiology* (5th edn.). Dubugne, IA: W. C. Brown.

Frankel F., Myatt R., Sugar C., Whitham, C., Gorospe, C. and Laugeson, E. (2010) "A randomized controlled study of parent-assisted children's friendship training with children having autism spectrum disorders." *Journal of Autism Developmental Disorders 40,* 7, 827–842.

Freed, J. and Parsons, L. (1997) *Right-brained Children in a Left-brained World: Unlocking the Potential of your ADD Child.* New York: Simon & Schuster.

Frumkin, H. (2001) "Beyond toxicity: human health and the natural environment." *American Journal of Preventative Medicine 20,* 3, 234–240.

Frumkin, H. and Eysenbach, M.E. (2007) "How cities use parks to improve public health." *American Planning Association: City Parks Forum,* 1–4.

Gaigg, S.B. and Bowler, D.M. (2007) "Differential fear conditioning in Asperger's syndrome: implication for an amygdala theory of autism." *Neuropsychologia 45,* 9, 2125–2134.

Gaines, K.S., Sancribrian, S. and Lock, R. (2011) *"The impact of classroom design on students with autism spectrum disorders."* Poster presentation at Autism Society's 42nd National Conference, Orlando, Florida, July 6–9.

Geen, R.G. (1978) "Effects of attack and uncontrollable noise on aggression." *Journal of Research in Personality 12,* 15–29.

Geen, R.G. and McCown, E.J. (1984) "Effects of noise on aggression and physiological arousal." *Motivation and Emotion 8,* 3, 231–241.

Gernsbacher, M.A., Dawson, M. and Goldsmith, H.H. (2005) "Three reasons not to believe in an autism epidemic." *Current Directions in Psychological Science 14,* 55–58.

Gershon, M. (1998) *The Second Brain.* New York: Harper Collins Publisher.

Gilbert, J.A., Krajmalnik-Brown, R., Porazinska, D.L., Weiss, S.J. and Knight, R. (2013) "Toward effective probiotics for autism and other neurodevelopmental disorders." *Cell 155*, 7, 1446.

Glaser, R. and Kiecolt-Glaser, J.K. (2005) "Stress-induced immune dysfunction: implications for health." *Nature Reviews Immunology 5*, 243–251.

Glass, D.C. and Singer, J.E. (1972a) *Urban Stress: Experiments on Noise and Social Stressors.* New York: Academic Press.

Glass, D.C. and Singer, J.E. (1972b) "Behavioral after effects of unpredictable and uncontrollable aversive events." *American Scientist 60*, 457–465.

Goldapple, K., Segal, Z., Garson, C. and Lau, M. *et al.* (2004) "Modulation of cortical-limbic pathways in major depression: treatment-specific effects of cognitive behavior therapy." *Archives of General Psychiatry 61*, 1, 34–41.

Gomez, P. and Danuser, B. (2007) "Relationships between musical structure and psychophysiological measures of emotion." *Emotion 7*, 2, 377–387.

Gomez-Pinilla, F. (2011) "The combined effects of exercise and foods in preventing neurological and cognitive disorders." *Preventative Medicine 52*, 1, S75–S80.

Grandin, T. (1984) "My experiences as an autistic child." *Journal of Orthomolecular Psychiatry 13*, 166–169.

Grandin, T. (2006) *Thinking in Pictures and Other Reports from My Life with Autism* (2nd edn.). London: Bloomsbury.

Green, S.A., Rudie, J.D., Colich, N.L. and Shirinyan, D. *et al.* (2013) "Overreactive brain responses to sensory stimuli in youth with autism spectrum disorders." *Journal of American Academy of Child and Adolescent Psychiatry 52*, 1158–1172.

Greer, S.M., Goldstein, A.N. and Walker, M.P. (2013) "The impact of sleep deprivation on food desire in the human brain." *National Communication 4*, 2259.

Groden, J., Cautela, J.R., Prince, S. and Berryman, J. (1994) "The Impact of Stress and Anxiety on Individuals with Autism and Developmental Disabilities." In E. Schopler and G.B. Mesibov (eds.) *Behavioral Issues in Autism.* New York: Plenum Press.

Gupta, S., Ellis, S., Ashar, F. and Moes, A. *et al.* (2014) "Transcriptome analysis reveals dysregulation of innate immune response genes and neuronal activity-dependent genes in autism." *Nature Communications 5*, 5748.

Hannah, L. (2001) *Teaching Young Children with Autistic Spectrum Disorders: A Practical Guide for Parents and Staff in Mainstream Schools and Nurseries.* London: National Autistic Society.

Hillier, A., Greher, G., Poto, N. and Dougherty, M. (2011) "Positive outcomes following participation in a music intervention for adolescents and young adults on the autism spectrum." *Psychology of Music 40*, 2, 201–215.

Hsiao, E.Y., McBride, S.W., Hsien, S. and Gil, S. *et al.* (2013) "Microbiota modulate behavioral and physiological abnormalities associated with neurodevelopmental disorders." *Cell 155*, 7, 1451–1463.

Humphreys, S., Gringras, P., Blair, P.S. and Scott, N. *et al.* (2014) "Sleep patterns in children with autistic spectrum disorders: a prospective study." *Archives of Disease in Childhood 99*, 2, 114–118.

Ingersoll, B., Walton, J., Carlsen, D. and Hamlin, T. (2013) "Social intervention for adolescents with autism and significant intellectual disability: initial efficacy of reciprocal imitation training." *American Journal of Intellectual Disabilities 118*, 4, 247–261.

Jeste, S.S. (2011) "The neurology of autism spectrum disorders." *Current Opinion in Neurology 24*, 2, 132–139.

Jolliffe, T., Lansdown, R. and Robinson, C. (1992) "Autism: a personal account." *Communication 6*, 3, 12–19.

Just, M.A., Cherkassky, V.L., Keller, T.A., Kana, R.K. and Minshew, N.J. (2007) "Functional and anatomical cortical underconnectivity in autism: evidence from an FMRI study of an executive function task and corpus callosum morphometry." *Cerebral Cortex 17*, 4, 951–961.

Kaiser Family Foundation (2010) *Generation M2: Media in the Lives of 8- to 18-Year-Olds.* Menlo Park, CA: Henry J. Kaiser Family Foundation.

Kanner, L. (1943) "Autistic disturbances of affective contact." *Nervous Child: Journal of Psychopathology, Psychotherapy, Mental Hygiene, and Guidance of the Child 2*, 217–250.

Katz, D.L., Katz, C.S., Treu, J.A. and Reynolds, J. *et al.* (2011) "Teaching healthful food choices to elementary school students and their parents: the Nutritional Detective program." *Journal of School Health 81*, 1, 21–28.

Kern, L., Koegel, R.L. and Dunlap, G. (1984) "The influence of vigorous versus mild exercise on autistic stereotyped behaviors." *Journal of Autism and Developmental Disorders 14*, 1, 57–67.

Kestenbaum, R., Farber, E.A. and Sroufe, L.A. (1989) "Individual differences in empathy among preschoolers: relation to attachment history." *New Directions for Child and Adolescent Development 1989*, 44, 51–64.

Kim, J., Wigram, T. and Gold, C. (2009) "Emotional, motivational and interpersonal responsiveness of children with autism in improvisational music therapy." *Autism 13*, 4, 389–409.

Kim, J.A., Szatmari, P., Bryson, S.E., Streiner, D.L. and Wilson, F.J. (2000) "The prevalence of anxiety and mood problems among children with autism and Asperger syndrome." *Autism 4*, 117–132.

Kim, Y.S., Leventhal, B.L., Koh, Y.J. and Fombonne, E. *et al.* (2011) "Prevalence of autism spectrum disorders in a total population sample." *American Journal of Psychiatry 168*, 9, 904–912.

Koenig, K.P., Buckley-Reen, A. and Garg, S. (2012) "Efficacy of the Get Ready to Learn Yoga program among children with autism spectrum disorders: a pretest-posttest control group design." *American Journal of Occupational Therapy 66*, 5, 538–546.

Kohane, I.S., McMurry, A., Weber, G. and MacFadden, D. *et al.* (2012) "The co-morbidity burden of children and young adults with autism spectrum disorders." *PLoS ONE 7*, 4, e33224.

Kondracki, N.L. (2012) "The link between sleep and weight gain: research shows poor sleep quality raises obesity and chronic disease risk." *Today's Dietitian 14*, 6, 48.

Krakowiak, P., Goodlin-Jones, B., Hertz-Picciotto, I., Croen, L.A. and Hansen, R.L. (2008) "Sleep problems in children with autism spectrum disorders, developmental delays, and typical development: a population-based study." *Journal of Sleep Research 17*, 197–206.

Kramer, A.F. and Erickson, K.I. (2007) "Capitalizing on cortical plasticity: influence of physical activity on cognition and brain function." *Trends in Cognitive Science 11*, 8, 342–348.

Kushki, A., Drumm, E., Pla Mobarak, M., Tanel, N. and Dupuis, A. (2013) "Investigating the autonomic nervous system response to anxiety in children with autism spectrum disorders." *PLOS One 8*, 4., e59730.

Kuypers, L. (2011) *Zones of Regulation.* San Jose, CA: Think Social Publishing.

Lackney, J. (2003) "Architecture of schools: the new learning environment." *Children, Youth and Environments 13*, 1.

Lang, R., Koegel, L.K., Ashbaugh, K., Regester, A., Ence, W. and Smith, W. (2010a) "Physical exercise in children with autism spectrum disorders: a systematic review." *Research in Autism Spectrum Disorders 4*, 565–576.

Lang R., Regester, A., Lauderdale, S., Ashbaugh, K. and Haring, A. (2010b) "Treatment of anxiety in autism spectrum disorders using cognitive behaviour therapy: a systematic review." *Developmental Neurorehabilitation 13*, 1, 53–63.

Lavelle, T.A., Weinstein, M.C., Newhouse, J.P. Munir, K., Kuhlthau, K.A. and Prosser, L.A. (2014) "Economic burden of childhood autism spectrum disorders." *Pediatrics, 133*, 3, e520-e529.

LeBlanc, L.A. and Coates, A.M. (2003) "Using video modeling and reinforcement to teach perspective-taking skills to children with autism." *Journal of Applied Behavior Analysis 36*, 2, 253–257.

Leyfer, O.T., Folstein, S.E., Bacalman, S. and Davis, N.O. *et al.* (2006) "Comorbid psychiatric disorders in children with autism: interview development and rates of disorders." *Journal of Autism and Developmental Disorders 36*, 849–861.

Looking Up (2013) "Feeding problems in autism." *Looking Up: The Monthly International Autism Magazine 5*, 8, 15-16.

Ludwig, D.S., Peterson, K.E. and Gortmaker, S.L. (2001) "Relation between consumption of sugar-sweetened drinks and childhood obesity: a prospective, observational analysis." *Lancet 357*, 505–508.

Malik, V.S., Willett, W.C. and Hu, F.B. (2009) "Sugar-sweetened beverages and BMI in children and adolescents: reanalyses of a meta-analysis." *American Journal of Clinical Nutrition 89*, 438–439.

Malik, V.S., Popkin, B.M., Bray, G.A., Despres, J.P., Willett, W.C. and Hu, F.B. (2010) "Sugar-sweetened beverages and risk of metabolic syndrome and Type 2 diabetes." *Diabetes Care 33*, 2477–2483.

Malow, B.A. and McGrew, S. (2008) "Sleep disturbances and autism." *Sleep Medicine Clinics 3*, 479–488.

Mayer, E.A. and Tillisch, K. (2011) "The brain-gut axis in abdominal pain syndromes." *Annual Review of Medicine 6*, 381–396.

Mazurek, M.O., Vasa, R.A., Kalb, L.G. and Kanne, S.M. *et al.* (2013) "Anxiety, sensory over-responsivity, and gastrointestinal problems in children with autism spectrum disorders." *Journal of Abnormal Child Psychology 41*, 1, 165–176.

McClannahan, L.E. and Krantz, P.J. (1997) "In Search of Solutions to Prompt Dependence: Teaching Children with Autism to Use Photographic Activity Schedules." In E.M. Pinkston and D.M. Baer (eds) *Environment and Behavior*. Boulder, CO: Westview Press.

McElhanon, B.O., McCracken, C., Karpen, S. and Sharp, W.G. (2014) "Gastrointestinal symptoms in autism spectrum disorders: a meta-analysis." *Pediatrics 133*, 5, 872–883.

McEwen, B. and Lasley, E. (2002) *The End of Stress As We Know It*. Washington, DC: Joseph Henry Press.

McGimsey, J.K. and Favell, J.E. (1988) "The effects of increased physical exercise on disruptive behaviors in retarded persons." *Journal of Autism and Developmental Disorders 18*, 167–179.

Michael Singer Studio and The Center for Discovery (2014) *A new model for shared housing: Individuals with autism spectrum conditions: A population positively affected by sustainable practices*. Available at www.michaelsinger. com/#/shared-living-for-adults-with-autism/, accessed on 03 March, 2014.

Moore, K.S. (2013) "A systematic review on the neural effects of music on emotion regulation: Implications for music therapy practice." *Journal of Music Therapy Practice 50*, 3, 198–242.

Mott, M.S., Robinson, D.H., Walden, A., Burnette, J. and Rutherford, A. (2012) "Illuminating the effects of dynamic lighting on student learning." *Sage Open 1–9*. Available at http://sgo.sagepub.com/content/2/2/2158244012445585, accessed on 19 August, 2015.

Mozaffarian, D., Katan, M.B., Ascherio, A., Stampfer, M.J. and Willett, W.C. (2006) "Trans fatty acids and cardiovascular disease." *New England Journal of Medicine 354*, 15, 1601–1613.

Nader-Grosbois, N. and Mazzone, S. (2014) "Emotion regulation, personality and social adjustment in children with autism spectrum disorders." *Psychology 5*, 1750–1767.

National Institute of Health (2014) *Interagency Autism Coordinating Committee*. Available at http://iacc.hhs.gov/, accessed on 11 February, 2015.

Naviaux, R.K., Zolkipli, Z., Wang, L. and Nakayama, T. *et al.* (2013) "Antipurinergic therapy corrects the autism-like features in the poly(IC) mouse model." *PLoS ONE 8*, 3, e57380.

New York Daily News (2013) "Son saved by Scrooge: 'Carol' Center Heals Troubled Soul." 20 December.

New York Daily News (2014) "Dance Dynamo: Prom Shows Just How Far Autistic Queens Man Has Come." 20 May.

New York Times, The (2015) "Losing the Home He's Known." New York Edition, 1 February, p. MB1.

O"Neill, J.L. (1998) *Through the Eyes of Aliens: A Book About Autistic People.* London: Jessica Kingsley Publishers.

Oriel, K.N., George, C.L., Peckus, R. and Semon, A. (2011) "The effects of aerobic exercise on academic engagement in young children and autism spectrum disorders." *Pediatric Physical Therapy 23*, 2, 187–193.

Perica, M.M. and Delas, I. (2011) "Essential fatty acids and psychiatric disorder." *Nutrition in Clinical Practice 26*, 409–425.

Piochon, C., Kloth, A.D., Grasselli, G. and Titley, H.K. *et al.* (2014) "Cerebellar plasticity and motor learning deficits in a copy-number variation mouse model of autism." *Nature Communications 5*, 5586.

Prior, M. and Ozonoff, S. (1998) "Psychological Factors in Autism." In F.R. Volkmar (ed.) *Autism and Pervasive Developmental Disorders.* Cambridge: Cambridge University Press.

Purdy, J. (2013) "Chronic physical illness: A psychopshysiological approach for chronic physical illness." *The Yale Journal of Biology and Medicine 86*, 1, 15-28.

Ramirez, G. and Beilock, S.L. (2011) "Writing about testing worries boosts exam performance in the classroom." *Science 331*, 211–213.

Ratey, J. (2008) *SPARK: The Revolutionary New Science of Exercise and the Brain.* New York: Little, Brown, and Company.

Ratey, J. and Sands, S. (1986) "The concept of noise." *Psychiatry 49*, 290–297.

Ratey, J. and Manning, R. (2014) *Go Wild: Free Your Body and Mind from the Afflictions of Civilization.* New York: Little, Brown, and Company.

Rea, M.S. (2000) *The IESNA Lighting Handbook: Reference and Application* (9th edn.). New York: Illuminating Engineering Society of North America.

Rechtschaffen, S. (1996) *Time Shifting: Create More Time to Enjoy Your Life.* New York: Broadway Books.

Richardson, A.J. (2003) "The importance of omega-3 fatty acids for behavior, cognition and mood." *Nutrition and the Brain 47*, 2, 92–98.

Ring, H.A., Baron-Cohen, S., Wheelwright, S. and Williams, S.C.R. *et al.* (1999) "Cerebral correlates of preserved cognitive skills in autism: a functional MRI study of embedded figures task performance." *Brain 122*, 1305–1315.

Ross, B.M. (2009) "Omega-3 polyunsaturated fatty acids and anxiety disorders." *Prostaglandins, Leukotrienes and Essential Fatty Acids 81*, 5–6, 309–312.

Samson, A.C., Huber, O. and Gross, J.J. (2012) "Emotion regulation in Asperger's syndrome and high-functioning autism." *Emotion 12*, 4, 659–665.

Sapolsky, R.M. (1998) *Why Zebras Don't Get Ulcers: An Updated Guide to Stress, Stress-Related Diseases, and Coping.* New York: W.H. Freeman and Co.

Sapolsky, R.M. (2004) *Why Zebras Don't Get Ulcers: An Updated Guide to Stress, Stress-Related Diseases, and Coping.* New York: Holt, Henry, and Co., Inc.

Schieve, L.A., Gonzales, V., Boulet, S.L. and Visser, S.N. *et al.* (2011) "Concurrent medical conditions and health care use and needs among children with learning and behavioral disabilities: National Health Interview Survey, 2006–2010." *Research in Developmental Disabilities 33*, 467–476.

Schoen, S.A., Miller, L.J., Brett-Green, B. and Hepburn, S. *et al.* (2008) "Psychophysiology in children with autism spectrum disorder." *Research in Autism Spectrum Disorders 2*, 3, 417–429.

Scholastic Inc. (2011) *The Mind-Up Curriculum: Brain-focused Strategies for Learning – and Living.* New York: Scholastic.

Schunk, D.H. and Zimmerman, B.J. (2007) "Influencing children's self-efficacy and self-regulation of reading and writing through modeling." *Reading and Writing Quarterly 23*, 7–25.

Selye, H. (1936) "A syndrome produced by diverse nocuous agents." *Nature 138*, 32.

Selye, H. (1955) "Stress and disease." *Science 122*, 625–631.

Shabha, G. (2006) "An assessment of the impact of the sensory environment on individuals" behaviour in special needs schools." *Facilities 24*, 1/2, 31–42.

Spratt, E.G., Nicholas, J.S., Brady, K.T., Carpenter, L.A. *et al.* (2012) "Enhanced cortisol response to stress in children with autism." *Journal of Autism and Developmental Disorders 42*, 1, 75–81.

Stein, L., Lane, C., Williams, M., Dawson, M., Polido, J. and Cermak, S. (2014) "Physiological and behavioral stress and anxiety in children with autism spectrum disorders during routine oral care." *BioMed Research International*, Article ID 694876.

Stokes, S. (2003) *National Association of Special Education Teachers. Autism Spectrum Disorders Series.* "Structured Teaching: Strategies for Supporting Students with Autism?" under a contract with CESA 7 and funded by a discretionary grant from the Wisconsin Department of Public Instruction. Available at www.specialed.us/autism/structure/str10.htm, accessed on 10 October, 2014.

Stone, N.J. and English, A.J. (1998) "Task type, posters, and workspace color on mood, satisfaction, and performance." *Journal of Environmental Psychology 18*, 175–185.

Storch, E.A., Lewin, A.B., Colier, A.B. and Arnold, E. *et al.* (2015) "A randomized control trial of cognitive-behavioral therapy versus treatment as usual for adolescents with autism spectrum disorders and comorbid anxiety." *Depression and Anxiety 21*, 174–181.

Tomanik, S., Harris, G.E. and Hawkins, J. (2004) "The relationship between behaviors exhibited by children with autism and maternal stress." *Journal of Intellectual & Developmental Disabilities 29*, 16–26.

Tononi, G. and Cirelli, C. (2014) "New hypothesis on why we sleep." *Scientific American Magazine 309*, 2, 34–39.

Ulrich, R.S. (1984) "View through window may influence recovery from surgery." *Science 22*, 420–421.

Ulrich, R.S., Simons, R.F., Losito, B.D., Fiorito, E., Miles, M.A. and Zelson, M. (1991) "Stress recovery during exposure to natural and urban environments." *Journal of Environmental Psychology 11*, 3, 201–230.

United States Department of Health and Human Services (2010) *Healthy People*. Washington, DC: US Government Printing Office.

United States Senate: Health, Education, Labor, and Pensions Committee. *Dangerous use of seclusion and restraints in schools remains widespread and difficult to remedy: A review of ten cases.* Majority Committee Staff Report. February 12, 2014.

Urry, H.L. (2010) "Seeing, thinking, and feeling: Emotion-regulating effects of gaze-directed cognitive reappraisal." *Emotion 10*, 1, 125–135.

Watters, R.G. and Watters, W.E. (1980) "Decreasing self-stimulatory behavior with physical exercise in a group of autistic boys." *Journal of Autism and Developmental Disorders 10*, 4, 379–387.

Webb, S.J., Jones, E.J.H., Merkle, K. and Venema, K. *et al.* (2011) "A developmental change in the ERP responses to familiar faces in toddlers with autism spectrum disorders versus typical development." *Child Development 82*, 6, 1868–1886.

Williams, D. (1996) *Autism, An Inside-Out Approach: An Innovative Look at the Mechanics of Autism and its Developmental Cousins.* London: Jessica Kingsley Publishers.

Williams, M.S. and Shellenberger, S. (1996) *How Does your Engine Run?: A Leaders Guide to the Alert Program for Self-regulation.* New Mexico: Therapy Works, Inc.

White, S.W., Oswald, D., Ollendick, T. and Scahill, L. (2009) "Anxiety in children and adolescents with autism spectrum disorders." *Clinical Psychology Review 29*, 3, 216–229.

Wood, J.J., Drahota, A., Sze, K., Har, K., Chiu, A. and Langer, D.A. (2009) "Cognitive behavioral therapy for anxiety in children with autism spectrum disorders: a randomized, controlled trial." *Journal of Child Psychology and Psychiatry 50*, 3, 224–234.

Wood, J.J., Ehrenreich-May, J., Alessandri, M., Fujii C., Renno, P. and Laugeson, E. *et al.* (2015) "Cognitive behavioral therapy for early adolescents with autism spectrum disorders and clinical anxiety: a randomized, controlled trial." *Behavior Therapy 46*, 7–19.

Woodyard, C. (2011) "Exploring the therapeutic effects of yoga and its ability to increase quality of life." *International Journal of Yoga 4*, 2, 49–54.

SUBJECT INDEX

AUTHOR INDEX